THE NEW
SEX
BIBLE
FOR WOMEN

A QUIVER BOOK

THE NEW SEX BIBLE FOR WOMEN

The Complete Guide to Sexual
Self-Awareness and Intimacy

AMIE HARWICK, M.A.

© 2015 Quiver

First published in the USA in 2015 by
Quiver, a member of
Quarto Publishing Group USA Inc.
100 Cummings Center
Suite 406-L
Beverly, MA 01915-6101
www.quiverbooks.com

The Publisher maintains the records relating to
images in this book required by 18 USC 2257.
Records are located at Rockport Publishers, Inc.,
100 Cummings Center, Suite 406-L, Beverly,
MA 01915-6101.

18 17 16 15 14   1 2 3 4 5

ISBN: 978-1-59233-641-8

Digital edition published in 2015
eISBN: 978-1-62788-185-2

Library of Congress Cataloging-in-Publication
Data available

Cover and book design by Burge Agency
Photography by Holly Randall
Image on page 21 courtesy of Shutterstock

Printed and bound in Hong Kong

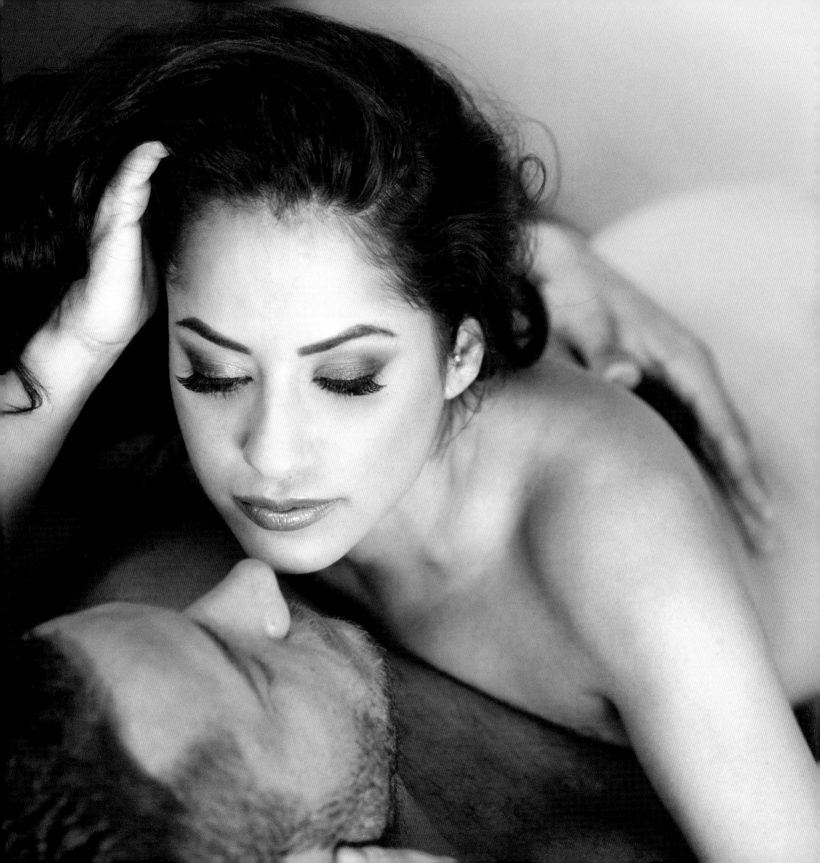

	Introduction	9
01	Your Body, Your Temple	13
02	Loving Your Sexual Life Span	33
03	Boosting Your Sexual Self-Esteem	55
04	The Brain: Your Most Powerful Sex Organ	71
05	Orgasms: Getting to the Big "O"	85
06	The Male Body: His Pleasure, Your Pleasure	99
07	Sex Positions: Poses That Boost Passion and Pleasure	113
08	Anal Sex: The Forbidden Fruit	135
09	Oral Sex: Be Great at Giving It— and Getting It	149
10	Sex Toys: Tools of the Trade	163
11	Alternative Lifestyles and Practices: Threesomes, BDSM, and Lots More	175
	Resources	184
	Index	187
	About the Author	190
	Acknowledgments	191

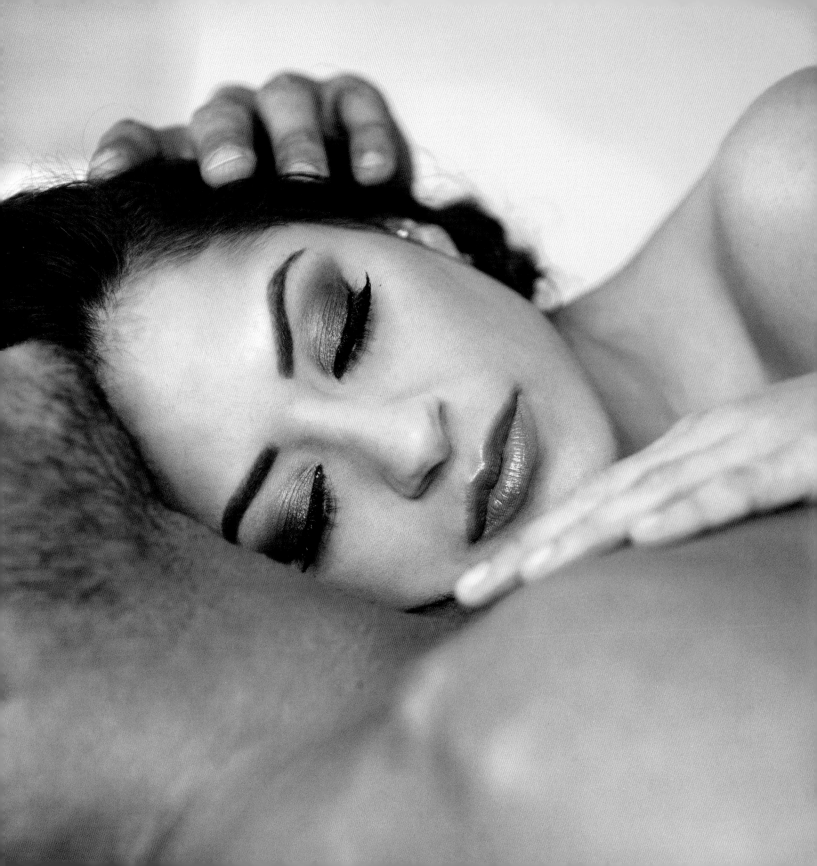

Introduction

You already know how unique you are as a person: you've got thousands of likes, dislikes, strengths, weaknesses, and quirks that make you *you*. Same goes for your sexual self: you've got your own needs and desires, and they're not the same needs as your sister's, your best friend's, or those of the woman sitting next to you on the subway. They're also different from those of your partner. That's why getting and staying in touch with your woman's body and your sexual self is so important: it's the first step on the path toward lifelong sexual fulfillment, sexual empowerment, and sexual pleasure. And guess what: as a sexual being, it's your right to have the sex you want—*when* you want it, and *how* you want it. It's true that, culturally, female sexuality has been dismissed, belittled, and even reviled—regardless of the fact that sexuality is a normal and natural part of any adult life. We're going to change all that. Your sexuality is yours to own, control, and indulge in—and it's time to celebrate that fact.

I'm Amie Harwick, and I'm a sex therapist. I'm here to help you have great sex, and—just as important—to love having it. And the best way to get started is to examine your own specific sexual needs. What are you curious about? What would you like to experiment with? What are you afraid of? What are your major turn-ons—and turn-offs? You might like to:

Do a little self-searching by writing in a journal. You're writing for you and you only, so go ahead and let it all out. Get racy: write down the most "out-there" fantasy you've ever had. Jot down your biggest fear—even if you think it'll sound silly. Writing down thoughts and feelings helps you acknowledge and process them.

Engage in thoughtful meditation. Set aside a while a few times a week to turn off the TV, your smartphone, and your laptop, and to think about your body and your sexual self. Let your mind wander. What's the best sexual experience you've ever had? Was it with a partner—or just yourself? What about the worst? How do you want to live your sexual life from this day forward?

Speak to a sex-positive therapist. (*Sex-positive* means that all legal and consensual sexuality is regarded as healthy and positive.) At first, talking about intimate things like sex and the way you feel about your own body to a "stranger" might feel a little weird. That's okay—it gets easier, and a supportive, sex-positive therapist can be a big help when it comes to embracing your own unique sexuality.

MIND-BLOWING SEX: IT'S ALL ABOUT YOU

Owning your sexuality also means being perceptive to cultural messages that conflict with your personal sexual empowerment. What does that mean? Well, the media and other implicit cultural messages often encourage women to believe that adult sexuality should focus on a man's fulfillment and orgasm. Even messages from the medical community don't seem to prioritize female sexual empowerment: the prevalence and visibility of Viagra and other male sexual-enhancement medications implies that sexuality, especially as you age, revolves around the male erection. Unfortunately, the sexual issues that women face as they age—such as an increased need for lubrication—haven't benefited from the same "normalizing" dialogue. The covers of women's magazines are strewn with bold, front-page proclamations, like "How to Blow His Mind in Bed" or "Tips to Please Him," instead of focusing on the woman's needs. It's no surprise, then, that so many women believe that *his* orgasm is at the center of the sexual experience: years of exposure to cultural messages like these tend to make us consciously—or unconsciously—place male sexual needs above our own. But it doesn't have to be this way. Sure, connective sex with a partner is great—but remember that having an orgasm doesn't require a partner at all. Ultimately, sex is a shared experience between two (or more) adults, and it's about mutual sexual pleasure; it doesn't revolve around male sexuality, unless you let it.

LET'S TALK (AND THINK) ABOUT SEX

Learning more about your own body and your own sexuality is key to having mind-blowing sex. Congratulations! You've already taken the first step by reaching for this book. Staying in touch with your sexual needs is a lifelong process—and it's a rewarding and fulfilling one. That said, it's important to reach out to trusted friends, a therapist, or other resources, if:

You feel sexually stuck. Has the sex in your relationship become routine and less fulfilling? The solution may be as simple as learning a few new techniques and focusing on communicating better with your partner.

You're coping with the changes that pregnancy can make to your sex life. As wonderful as it is, pregnancy means that your body is changing, and this can also mean physical discomfort and psychological insecurity. Normalizing your experience and learning alternate sex positions can help make sex just as hot as it was before you got pregnant.

You're dying to expand your sexual repertoire. None of us were given a comprehensive handbook when we lost our virginity (unfortunately). You've learned what you know about sex through your own experimentation, and, perhaps, from talking to friends. Reading about sex and watching erotica, for example, can inspire you and help you to try new techniques and skills.

You have never had an orgasm. Don't worry: you *can* have one. Most of the time, the biggest barriers to orgasming are lack of skills, anxiety, feeling pressured, or feeling uncomfortable with your own body. That's okay. Take your time, relax, and look for help if you need it.

You've never had an orgasm with a partner. Lots of women have difficulty orgasming with a partner but are able to climax during masturbation. This book will show you how to relax and ease into the experience of orgasming *à deux*, so that you don't always have to go it solo.

You think that vagina means "everything between your legs." Think again! Your vagina is the canal that leads to your uterus, while your vulva is the external area between your legs. Knowing your lady parts is the most important thing when it comes to knowing your sexual self.

Once you've started to make mindful choices like these about your sexual self, you'll start to feel—and act—more sexually empowered. You'll be able to make healthy, educated choices regarding sex partners, and you'll find that you can gain sexual satisfaction either with a partner or on your own. Sexually empowered women often work to support and encourage other women through writing or education, or simply by lending an empathic ear to female friends. As the saying goes, the personal is political, so as you become sexually empowered, you change the lives of the women around you as well as your own.

START YOUR SEXUCATION

The New Sex Bible for Women is your guide on your journey to sexual empowerment. It's packed with everything you need to know to experience great sex, from a few woman-to-woman anatomy lessons to kinkier ways to have fun, like experimenting with group sex, anal sex, erotica, and sex toys. (If a technique piques your interest, check out the resource section at the back of this book for a list of websites, books, and films that'll help you explore it.) Rest assured that everything you'll read here is written from the perspective of a sex-positive feminist therapist who's on your side 110%. Finally, while this book is geared primarily toward heterosexual women, women of all sexual orientations will benefit from its woman-centered approach to loving your body and your sexuality.

Keep reading: the best sex of your life is just a few pages away.

—Amie Harwick, M.A.

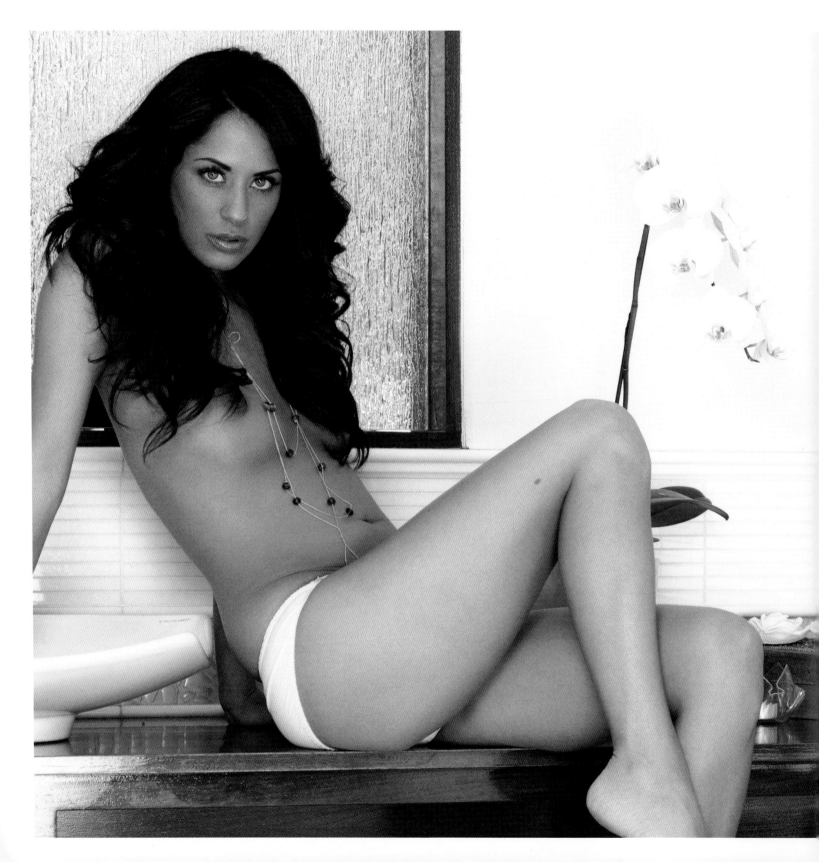

01 ♀ *Your Body, Your Temple*

Great sex starts with understanding your sexual anatomy. In this chapter I'll teach you to love those powerful erogenous zones that are your breasts, and you'll take Vagina 101, a quick refresher course that'll put you in touch with the anatomy and functions of your lady parts. You'll also learn the truth about the fabled G-spot (here's a hint: it's real!). And, just in case you've forgotten, there's nothing more important than your own sexual health, so I'll remind you how to stay safe by protecting yourself against sexually transmitted infections (STIs) and by choosing the right birth control option for you. Get ready to make your body your best friend.

GREAT SEX STARTS WITH YOU

First things first. Knowing and loving your body inside and out—both literally and figuratively—is the very first step on the journey to great sex. Just like anything else you value as sacred, it's important to honor your body by giving it the time and attention it takes to know it well. If you're more than a little mystified by yours, don't worry: lots of women aren't on very intimate terms with their own sexual parts. The structure of women's sexual anatomy is tucked away neatly between our legs, and isn't physically (or culturally) available to us on a regular basis. Men, on the other hand, experience their sexual

kinesthetic awareness very differently. Due to the structure of his body, a man is able to see his penis every day, when he changes his clothes, urinates, or masturbates. It is always accessible to his eyes and hands. (It's even more culturally acceptable for a man to "adjust himself" in public than it is for a woman.) Women don't have the same access to most of their sexual anatomy, and so we have to be proactive when it comes to exploring our own bodies. And that's all part of the fun: understanding your basic sexual anatomy and its functions—and becoming aware of how you feel about your breasts, vagina, and other sexual parts—is one of the most important things you can do to ensure that you'll enjoy a lifetime of great sex.

BREASTS: BARING IT ALL

We've all got them—but what *are* breasts and what are they for? Well, the female breast is made of fifteen to twenty clusters of milk glands, or lobes. Each milk gland has a milk duct that leads to the nipple. Surrounding these milk glands are fatty tissue deposits that reside just under the skin of the breast. The areola, or the darkened area around the nipple, may contain small bumps, and may vary from woman to woman in size, shape, and color. During pregnancy, the breasts go through changes, such as swelling and preparation for milk production. Within two to three days of giving birth, the breasts lactate, or produce milk. To do so, the pituitary gland produces a protein called prolactin, which stimulates milk production, and releases a hormone called oxytocin, which encourages the ejection of milk from the nipple. Prolactin encourages a sense of gratification, while oxytocin—also known as the "love hormone"—produces feelings of warmth, affection, and a desire to bond.

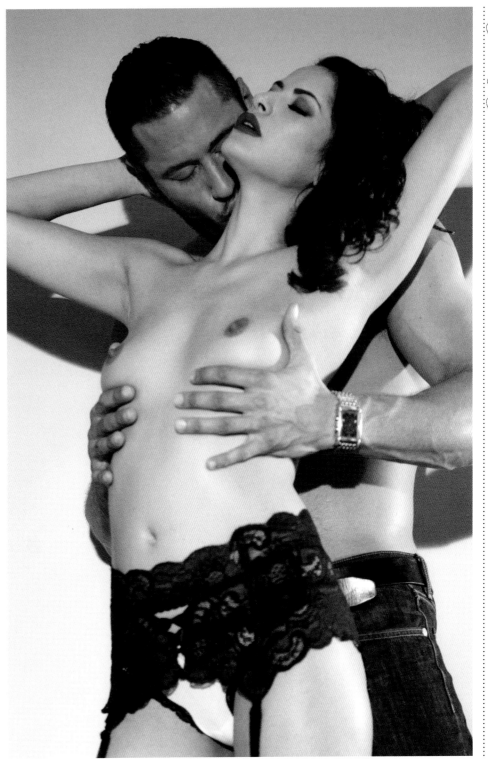

While breasts aren't technically sexual organs, they've been culturally associated with sex and they're the object of an overwhelming amount of cultural attention and criticism. Women with large breasts might feel that they're constantly being appraised or scrutinized, while women with small breasts can feel that they're unfeminine or even abnormal. The truth is, there's no such thing as "normal." Just like individual body shapes—and vaginal shapes and sizes—every woman has her own unique breast shape, size, and sensitivity level. And if your breasts are asymmetrical, know that you're in the majority: about 90% of women have at least a small degree of breast difference, whether it's in their shape or size. (In most cases, the left breast is slightly larger, which may be due to an increased blood flow from its proximity to the heart.) Also, as you age, you might find that your breasts tend to hang lower on your chest, with the nipple pointing downward. Known as breast ptosis, this is a natural progression. After all, everyone ages over time, and there's no avoiding gravity.

That said, it's true that breast perception is often attached to self-image in women. Due to the prevalent cultural emphasis on breasts, they can play a major role in the way a woman defines herself and her own femininity. When life circumstances such as aging or breast cancer occur, some women might find themselves questioning their self-image or sexual desirability, and even experiencing depression. It's important to remember that your breasts are a single aspect of your femininity—not its sum total.

And when it comes to breast shape and size, a recent study at the Victoria University of Wellington in New Zealand has shown that men don't necessarily think bigger is better, either. The study hypothesized that men would be more attracted to larger-breasted women, but its results demonstrated that, in fact, men responded equally to bare-chested women of all breast sizes. That means that men are simply attracted to breasts, period. In effect, desirable breast size varies among cultures. While some cultures

seem to gravitate toward fuller, larger breasts, others value smaller, perkier breasts, or breasts that hang downward. The moral of the story? Don't bother comparing your breasts to anyone else's. That's boring and counterproductive. It's far more worthwhile to love the beautiful breasts you've got.

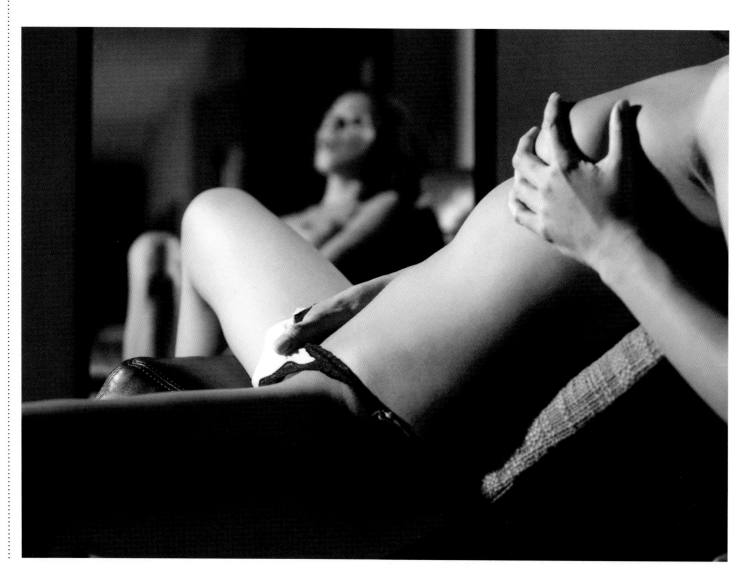

Plus, breasts can make hot sex even hotter. While your breasts aren't technically sexual organs, they're certainly part of your sexual experience. Because the breasts and nipples contain millions of sensitive nerve endings, they're powerful erogenous zones. When aroused, your nipples may harden, your breasts might swell, and, because nipple stimulation is received by the same part of the brain as genital stimulation, they can create uterine contractions, cause plenty of erotic pleasure, and even stimulate vaginal lubrication. That means that showing your breasts some love—or letting him do it—can be a huge part of self-pleasure, foreplay, sex, or a steamy make-out session. Next time you're getting it on with your partner, try these tips for making the most of your breasts:

Show him what you like. Lightly touch your breasts the way that you want him to touch them. He'll learn exactly what you want him to do, and he'll probably be hugely turned on by watching you.

Reach out. Take his hands and place them on your breasts. It's empowering to use your hands to show him exactly where—and how—you like to be stroked.

Pleasure spiked with pain. Go ahead and pinch, squeeze, flick, or twist your nipples—or ask him to do it for you. A little pain can be very pleasurable. (A little goes a long way, though: start out very gently to find out whether it's right for you.)

Get nailed. Have him lightly run his fingernails over your nipples. They're so sensitive that even the gentle pressure of his nails can be an incredible turn-on.

Bite me. Ask him to lightly bite your nipples—and to quickly follow up with a gentle kiss.

Go hot and cold. Temperature sensations can really drive you crazy. Get him to help you anoint your breasts and nipples with warming oils, or to tease them by brushing them with ice cubes.

Keep him hard. Stimulate his penis by using both your breasts and your hands. Place his penis between your breasts and use your hands to masturbate him.

Exploring what works for you when you're enjoying sex with your partner is great, but don't forget that your breasts are yours alone. Sure, breasts are functional: they can both feed babies and give you immense sexual pleasure. But your boobs don't belong to the doctors that squeeze them into cold mammograms, to the media, to your critical peers, or even to your lovers. They're all yours. Here's how to show them the love they deserve:

Get up close and personal. Stand in front of a mirror and look at your breasts. Examine them. Get to know them. What makes them special or different? Which parts of them do you love the most? Maybe it's your nipple size, your breast shape, or the way they feel so soft to the touch.

Feel the love. Surround yourself with breast-positive partners and friends. If your partner or a friend criticizes your breasts, it may be time for a direct conversation—or it may even be time to consider whether that person deserves a place in your life. If your partner isn't already complimenting your breasts, it's okay to ask him for a compliment. Ask him to tell you what he likes about them.

Give them a rubdown. Breasts have relatively thin skin and can be prone to dryness. Show them some love by giving them a quick massage with your favorite lotion. You'll love how soft and smooth they feel.

Stay healthy. It's a cliché, but it's true: preventive health is the best medicine. Give yourself regular breast self-exams, and be sure to talk to your doctor about any abnormalities you might have noticed.

VAGINA 101: A CRASH COURSE

Think everything between your legs is your vagina? Think again. Your vagina is just one of many lady parts that make up your sexual anatomy—and your sexual pleasure certainly doesn't begin and end with it. Didn't know that? Don't worry: historically, because the majority of medical and educational materials regarding female sexual anatomy were written by men, they tended to focus on the reproductive value of the female genitals rather than their potential for sexual pleasure. (Anatomic medical researchers of the sixteenth century left the clitoris out of anatomy texts altogether.) It's time to write the pleasure back in. The area around your vagina and vulva can be a veritable treasure trove of erotic pleasure. Let's go over the basics of your sexual anatomy—and take a quick refresher course in how to enjoy it.

THE EXTERNAL SEX ORGANS

The external female sex organs—also known as the vulva—include the mons, the labia majora, the labia minora, the clitoris, and the opening of the vagina.

The mons is the soft fatty tissue located over the public bone. The mons—sometimes called the pubic mound—becomes covered with hair during puberty. This area contains a wealth of nerve endings. Although many women rub the mons during masturbation, it's rarely depicted in adult films or magazines. Put the mons back on your sexual map: it's a highly sensitive area, and simply putting a little pressure or friction on it can lead to orgasm.

The labia majora, also called the outer lips, are two outer folds of skin covering the labia minora, clitoris, urinary meatus, and vaginal opening. The labia majora begin at the mons and continue between the legs, ending just above the anus. The labia majora can vary in appearance: in some women, they can be relatively flat, while in others, they may be thicker and more prominent. They darken during puberty, although the shade varies among individuals. Their main function is to cover and protect the sexual organs. The labia majora constitute another highly sensitive area. Just lightly tracing your fingers over the labia—or having your partner do it—can be highly arousing. If you use your fingers to part your labia majora, you'll see and feel a smaller, thinner set of "lips" called the labia minora (also called the inner lips). They're two folds of asymmetrical skin that cover the clitoris and the urinary and vaginal openings, and, like the labia majora, they can vary in terms of size, shape, and color. The labia minora start at the prepuce, or the clitoral hood, and they're dense with nerves, which means that having them touched, licked, or sucked is usually very pleasurable.

The prepuce is the piece of skin that covers and protects the clitoral shaft. In addition to being sensitive in itself, moving this clitoral hood up and down strokes the clitoris, and can lead to orgasm. Rubbing the prepuce is a way to bring yourself to orgasm while alone, or while having sex with your partner.

The most sexually sensitive organ in the female body is the clitoris, which is located below the mons and under the prepuce. The external round tip that's visible under the prepuce is called the glans; it's the sensitive head of the clitoris. Although only the tip of the clitoris is visible, this organ is actually a system of nerves, blood vessels, and tissues that extends inside the body. The shaft of the clitoris extends from the clitoral hood

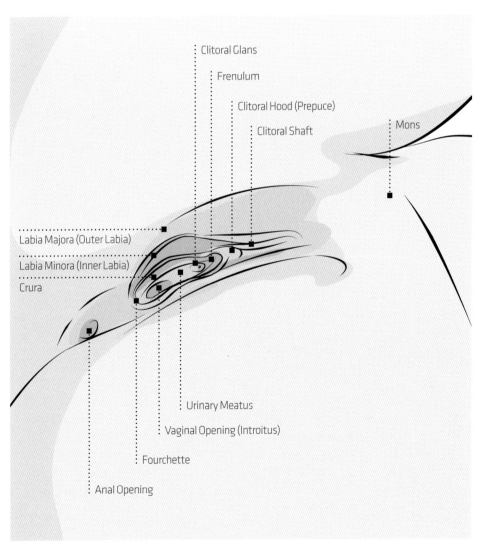

Clitoral Glans

Frenulum

Clitoral Hood (Prepuce)

Clitoral Shaft

Mons

Labia Majora (Outer Labia)

Labia Minora (Inner Labia)

Crura

Urinary Meatus

Vaginal Opening (Introitus)

Fourchette

Anal Opening

and contains erectile tissue, meaning that your clitoris will become erect and protrude when you are aroused.

The Bartholin's glands are located inside the labia minora, to the sides of the vaginal opening. They produce some of the fluid that keeps the vagina moist—although the majority of the lubrication that comes from arousal is produced deep inside the vagina. Moisture prevents the vulva and vagina from getting irritated, and makes penetration that much easier—and hotter.

Above the vaginal opening is the urinary meatus, or the urethral opening. The urinary meatus is the opening through which urine leaves the body. Below the urinary meatus is the introitus, which is the opening that leads to the vagina. In younger women, this opening may be partially covered by a hymen, a small piece of tissue that lies over the vaginal opening. Cultural presumptions imply that a hymen is present only in virgins, but the reality is that many women will have already broken their hymens prior to penis penetration. Accidents, self-exploration, and even walking and washing can cause the hymen to break. Because the hymen becomes thinner and smaller as a girl ages, there is often very little, if any, of the hymen left when she first experiences intercourse.

THE INTERNAL SEX ORGANS
The vagina is a muscular, elastic tube that's responsive to sexual arousal. It's located inside the body, past the vaginal opening. When there is nothing in the vaginal cavity, its walls may feel as if they have ridges. On average, the vagina is about 4 inches (10 centimeters) deep, with the potential to deepen and stretch: during arousal, the vagina can expand up to 200%, making it easy to accommodate most penis sizes. The well-known sex psychologists William Masters and Virginia Johnson (1966) found that the average depth of a vagina is 2.75–3 inches (7–8 centimeters), but that deepens to 4.3–4.7 inches (11–12 centimeters) when aroused. If you find that intercourse with a larger partner is painful, it might help to ensure that you are fully aroused before penetration.

Only the outer area of the vagina is sensitive; the inner parts of the vagina lack the many nerve endings of the outer parts.

The cervix is the lower neck of the uterus, which protrudes into the vagina, while the opening to the cervix is the os. Right above the cervix is the isthmus, which connects the body of the uterus to the cervix. The top of the uterus is called the fundus.

The uterus goes into the deeper part of the vagina. A muscular organ that contains an egg once fertilized, the uterus encases the fetus during pregnancy. The uterus is pear-shaped and about 3 inches (7.6 centimeters) long, and it's located above the vagina.

The walls of the uterus contain three layers: the outer layer, the perimetrium, is thin and acts as an outer cover. The middle layer, the myometrium, is comprised of thick and muscular tissue, and the innermost layer, the endometrium, contains glands and blood vessels. (When you menstruate each month, you shed the endometrium.) It's also responsible for providing nourishment to the fetus during pregnancy.

Two tubes on either side of the uterus, called the fallopian tubes, connect the uterus to the ovaries. The ovaries produce mature ova, or eggs, plus the female hormones estrogen and progesterone. The ovaries are about 1 inch (2.5 centimeters) long, and they contain capsules of cells called follicles, which contain cells that have the potential to develop into ova.

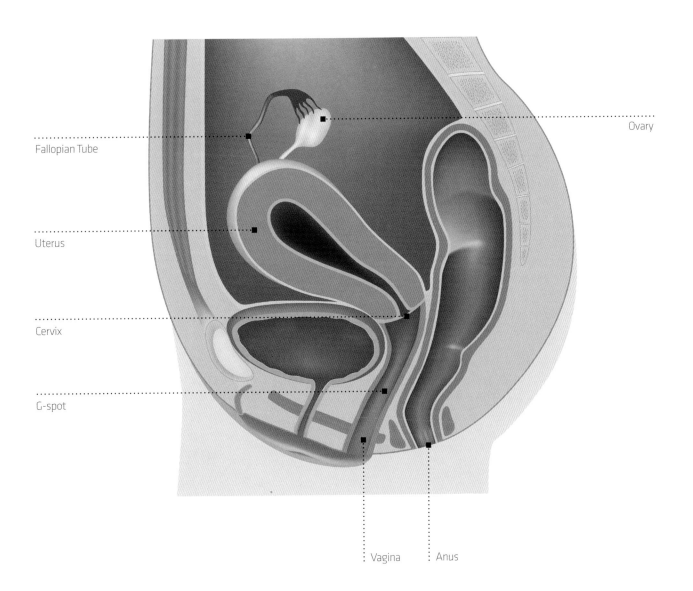

Fallopian Tube

Uterus

Cervix

G-spot

Ovary

Vagina

Anus

WHAT ABOUT THE G-SPOT?

The media makes much of the magical "G-spot." Both men's and women's magazines feature articles with advice on how to find it, and sex toys advertise a guarantee of G-spot stimulation. What they don't tell us is the important stuff, such as what the G-spot actually is, where to find it, and how it works. The fact is, the G-spot made its debut in 1981, when Beverly Whipple and John Perry published an article on it in the *Journal of Sex Research*, and named their newly discovered finding the Grafenberg spot, or the G-spot. Other researchers quickly added their voices: psychologist Josephine Sevely called it the *corpus spongiosus* and published this finding in her 1987 book *Eve's Secrets: A New Theory of Female Sexuality*, while others referred to the area as the urethral sponge.

To make a long story short, the G-spot is real: it's just been called by many different names over time. Basically, it's a spongy area made up of erectile tissue, located around the urethra, which, when aroused, prevents urination during sexual intercourse or other sexual activity. It's located behind the pubic bone and within the front wall of the vagina, and, while its exact size, shape, and location vary slightly in each woman, the fact is that every woman has one—which is a good thing, since the G-spot has more than a few sexual perks. When the area around the G-spot is aroused, it swells with blood, and its immense amount of nerve endings can be stimulated for serious pleasure—and it may even cause female ejaculation. (Yes, women can ejaculate, too!) Also, it surrounds the clitoral nerve, so stimulation of the clitoris may stimulate the G-spot as well, leaving you doubly aroused. Here's how to become acquainted with this fabled hotspot:

1. Wash your hands thoroughly. Be sure to have a water-based lubricant available, if needed.

2. While sitting or lying at an incline, insert your index finger into your vagina. If you insert your finger as far as possible, you should be able to feel the cervix.

3. Move your index finger in a "beckoning" gesture and, behind the upper wall of the vagina, you should feel a hard, walnut-shaped area. This is your G-spot.

4. Explore your G-spot and the area around it. Be aware of how the pressure of your finger feels on it. How sensitive is it?

5. Once you're on intimate terms with your G-spot, visit it frequently. Experiment with the different levels of pressure and find out what you like. Show your partner where it is—and don't be shy about showing him what you like.

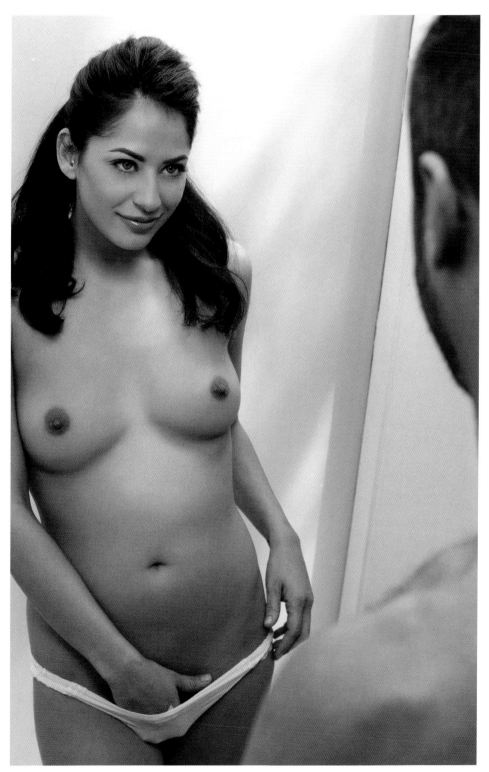

MEET YOUR VAGINA

Women's sexual parts aren't as visible to us on a daily basis as men's are. That means it takes a little extra time to get to know your vagina. But there's no need to contort yourself over a hand mirror to get a peek between your legs! Instead, follow these easy steps:

Grab a hands-free, standing mirror (some mirrors that are made for makeup application work really well here).

Make sure the room you're in is well lit, or bring a desk lamp near and angle it toward you to shed some light on the situation, so to speak.

Sit on the floor with the mirror in front of you and with your hips angled slightly upward. Once you're comfortable, use your fingers to spread your outer and then your inner labia.

Touch, stroke, and explore each part of your vagina. (Review our anatomy lesson in Vagina 101, if you like.) Pay attention to each part—labia minora, labia majora, mons, clitoris, whatever—and see what feels best for you. Notice the shape, color, texture, and size of all of your parts. Like the rest of you, it's completely unique. Your vagina is great because it's yours.

Another way to get to know your vagina is to draw it. (Relax: you don't have to be Picasso to reap the benefits of this exercise!) Still seated in front of your hands-free mirror, grab a piece of paper and any writing tool—pencil, pen, crayon, marker, or whatever's at hand. Draw what you see. By studying yourself, you'll notice parts of your sexual anatomy that you may not have been aware of before.

YOURSELF— ALWAYS

Your health is the most important thing in your world, and you've only got one vagina, so use it wisely. Take measures to protect yourself against sexually transmitted infections (STIs), and find an effective method of birth control that you're comfortable with. The reality is that STIs are all too common, and, thanks to biology, our bodies are constructed to get pregnant. Don't wait. Take control of your sexual health by:

1. Having a regular gynecological exam, and getting pap smears yearly. Ask your gynecologist questions and report any changes in your body you might have noticed.

2. Getting tested for STIs after every new partner, or yearly—whichever comes first. You should also get tested immediately if you feel that your monogamous relationship has been compromised by infidelity. Ask for an exam, cultures, and blood work. The fact is, if you take a casual attitude toward sexual safety, you could be placing your fertility at risk in the future.

3. Asking to see your partners' test results. Don't take their word for it: if a prospective partner won't show you his test results, keep your legs (and everything else) closed.

4. Buying condoms. Condoms are accessible, inexpensive, and easy to use. Lots of women are intimidated by the idea of buying them, but you need to get comfortable with it, stat, whether you're sexually active at the moment or not. Keep one pack at home and one in your purse.

5. Avoiding douching. Although it was common practice in years gone by, doctors today advise against it, because it can lead to infection and other issues.

6. Educating yourself on birth control methods, and consulting with your doctor on which are best for you.

BIRTH CONTROL AT A GLANCE

Speaking of birth control, here's a basic primer on available types of birth control. Using birth control isn't always fun, convenient, or "spontaneous," but with great power—and having sex *is* a great power!—comes great responsibility, and you can't neglect yours without risking serious consequences to yourself and your partner. Find the right type of birth control for you, and use it. Every single time.

Barrier methods involve the use of a physical barrier to prevent the exchange of body fluids. The most common form is the condom, which protects both partners from pregnancy as well as from sexually transmitted diseases. Others forms of the barrier method include the female condom, dental dams, and diaphragms.

Hormonal methods of birth control include the birth control pill, the patch, hormonal injections, and some intrauterine devices. Hormonal birth control prevents pregnancy but does not protect either partner against STIs. A nonhormonal, but internal, option of birth control is the nonhormonal IUD, which can be right for women who have trouble with the additional estrogen inherent in the hormonal choices.

Behavioral methods of birth control are far less reliable than barrier or hormonal methods. One so-called behavioral method is withdrawal, in which your partner pulls out before ejaculation. This method hardly deserves the name birth control, since the sperm in his preejaculate can still get you pregnant—even if he does pull out in time. So whatever you do, *don't* rely on withdrawal as a birth control method. Then there are fertility awareness methods, which involve having sex only at certain "safe" times of the month based on your ovulation cycle. You really need to be in touch with your body if you're going to try this kind of "rhythm" method, since it can involve monitoring your body temperature, knowing your menstrual cycle to the day, and checking your cervical mucus. So if you're a little squeamish about these things, it might be better to choose another form of birth control. Behavioral methods are best used in conjunction with another method of birth control. On their own, they're no more than an attempt at pregnancy prevention, and, of course, they don't protect either partner against STIs.

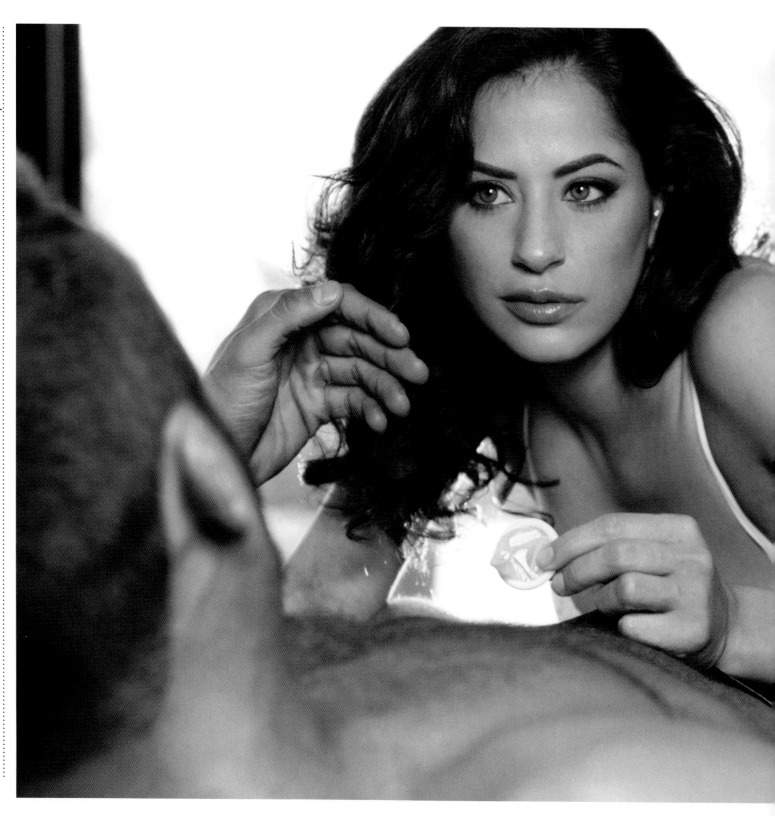

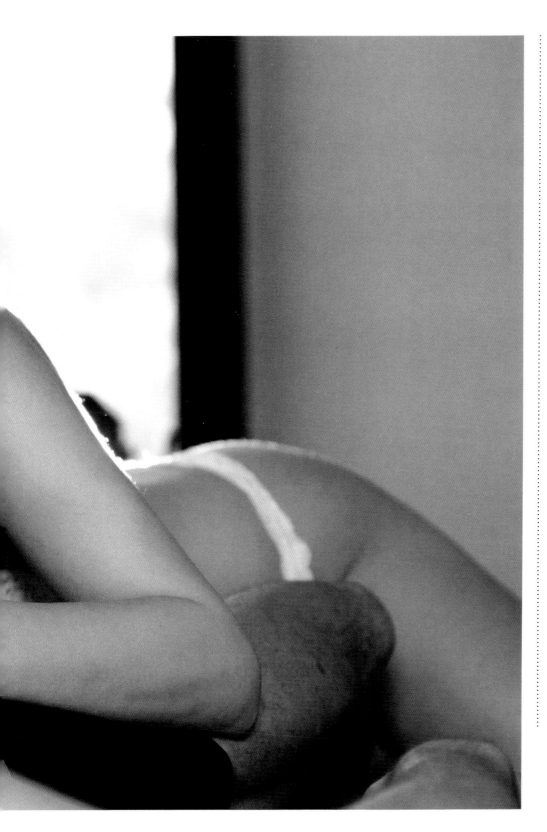

HOW TO PUT ON A CONDOM IN A FEW EASY STEPS

Condoms really are simple to use once
you've had a little practice.
Here's a quick usage guide:

Unwrap. Gently tear open the condom packet.
Be sure not to rip the condom itself. Watch
out for sharp fingernails or jewelry.

Pinch the tip. If there's any air in the tip of
the condom, squeeze it out before putting
it on. Air bubbles can cause condoms to
tear during sex.

Place the condom on the head of his penis,
then lightly and carefully unroll the condom
fully over the penis's shaft. Leave a little room
at the top for the semen.

Having trouble? If you're having trouble
unrolling the condom, check to see whether
it's inside out. If it is, start again with a fresh
condom. Don't turn it over and begin again
because his lubrication or precum can have
enough sperm to get you pregnant
and/or carry an STI.

Avoid using petroleum jelly or non-water-
based lubricants, because they can cause
condoms to break.

Pull out carefully. When he's pulling out, make
sure you or he holds the base of the condom
tightly so no semen spills out.

Dispose of the condom hygienically by
throwing it out. (Don't flush it down the
toilet.)

VAGINAL ISSUES AND CONCERNS

Just as they can impact the rest of your body, medical and psychological issues can affect your vagina. It's a sensitive area, and its balance can be disrupted by simple things like hormonal fluctuations, poor nutrition, lack of sleep, having unprotected sex, or new medications. (Contact your doctor right away if you experience symptoms such as vaginal bleeding, cramping, white discharge, or foul odors.) Sometimes, the source of vaginal discomfort isn't an infection, an STI, or lifestyle changes. Vaginismus is an unconscious vaginal contraction that occurs when something—a penis, a tampon, anything—approaches the vaginal opening. Its source might be physical: it can be caused by an issue with the muscles surrounding the vaginal area. It can also be caused by psychological issues, such as trauma or stress. If you have vaginismus, your sex-positive doctor will be able to recommend the right treatment for you, depending on its cause.

NAME	SYMPTOMS	CAUSE	TREATMENT	PREVENTION
Yeast infection	Thick white discharge that may resemble cottage cheese; itching and burning; swelling; pain during intercourse.	Caused by the introduction of new yeast or an imbalance in the types of bacteria inside your vagina, possibly due to having sex with a new partner. This imbalance can also be caused by antibiotics.	Over-the-counter treatment creams are available, but it's best to be examined by a doctor in order to rule out other types of infections. An oral treatment for yeast infections is also available through your doctor.	Eat foods that are rich in acidophilus, the good bacteria that exists in your vagina and digestive tract. Try foods like yogurt, whole wheat, tomatoes, onions, garlic, and bananas—or take acidophilus supplements. Wear breathable fabrics next to your body, such as cotton. Limit the time you spend in bubble baths, and try to reduce overall stress levels.
Urinary tract infection (UTI)	Pain during urination; blood or a foul odor in your urine.	Can occur naturally, or as a result of bacteria being pushed into the urethra during sex.	Antibiotics.	Urinate immediately after sex. Shower before and after sex, and use condoms.
Bacterial vaginosis (BV)	A fishy odor; white discharge; pain during urination. Sometimes no symptoms are present at all.	Can be sexually transmitted or can occur naturally.	Antibiotics.	BV can be prevented by use of condoms and good hygiene.
Trichinosis	Green or yellow discharge and a strong smell.	Parasite that is passed sexually.	Antibiotics.	Use condoms.
Gonorrhea and chlamydia	Similar to a yeast infection or urinary tract infection: burning during urination; discharge. Symptoms may not appear at all.	Sexually transmitted bacterial infections.	Antibiotics. If left untreated, gonorrhea and chlamydia can cause damage such as pelvic inflammatory disease.	Use condoms.
Syphilis	Sores or chancres on outer genitals or inside the vagina; swelling of lymph nodes.	Sexually transmitted bacterial infection.	Antibiotics.	Use condoms.

NAME	SYMPTOMS	CAUSE	TREATMENT	PREVENTION
Hepatitis A	Symptoms may take up to three months to develop and can include abdominal pain, dark urine, nausea, and joint pain.	Not technically an STI, but can be transmitted by anal contact during sex, or by foods that have touched infected tableware.	In most cases, hepatitis A goes away on its own without support from a physician.	Wash your hands regularly and thoroughly throughout the day. Contact your doctor if your partner has hepatitis A. Avoid eating in restaurants with poor sanitation, and never eat undercooked shellfish.
Hepatitis B	Chronic fatigue; yellowing of the skin or the whites of the eyes; fever; nausea or vomiting. However, symptoms may not appear at all.	Sexually transmitted virus.	While hepatitis B usually resolves on its own without support from a physician, some people develop a chronic hepatitis B infection, which can cause more severe issues such as liver damage and risk of liver cancer.	Use condoms, do not share razors or toothbrushes, and be sure to frequent clean and reputable tattoo or piercing shops only.
Hepatitis C	Fatigue, mild cognitive issues, liver damage. Often no symptoms appear for decades.	Not sexually transmitted, but can be transmitted through blood via shared needles or personal care items.	Avoid alcohol and certain medications; get vaccinated for hepatitis A and B. Treatment can also include antiviral medication.	Avoid sharing needles and personal care items, and see your doctor for education if your partner has been diagnosed.
Genital herpes	Blister-like sores around the mouth, anus, and genital area. However, symptoms may not appear at all.	Sexually transmitted virus.	Treatment includes repressive medication.	Use condoms.
Human papilloma virus (HPV)	Genital warts of varying sizes and shapes.	Sexually transmitted virus that has a few strains; some strains of HPV have been linked to cervical cancer.	Treatment for warts includes freezing and surgical removal.	Use condoms.
HIV/AIDS	No symptoms appear until about ten years after infection.	Sexually transmitted virus.	Prescription treatments for maintenance only; no cure available.	Use condoms.

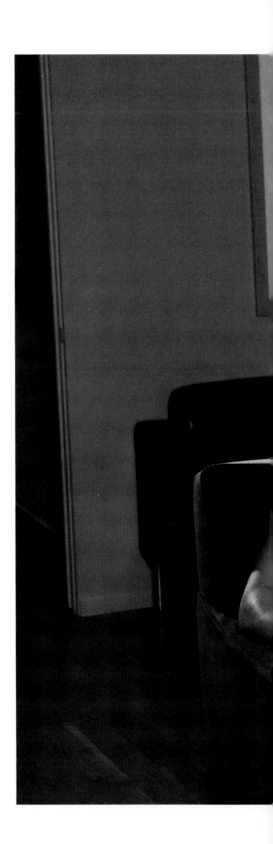

LOVE THE ONE YOU'VE GOT

Your body makes you the woman you are—and that means your body is beautiful. Its shape and size are uniquely your own, and it's yours to love, understand, and protect. Your breasts, vagina, and vulva are capable of giving you intense pleasure, and, what's more, they're seriously powerful, since they make it possible for you to give birth to other human beings. And they belong to you and you alone. When it comes to getting the great sex you deserve, knowing and loving your body inside and out is the first step. Of course, your body and your sexual needs will change over your lifetime. Read on to find out how to enjoy every minute of it.

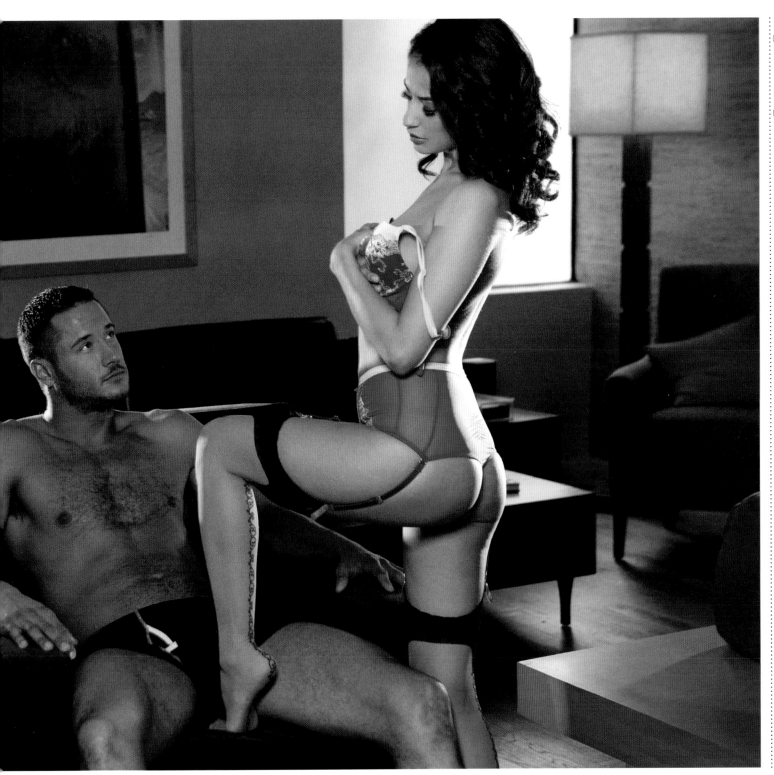

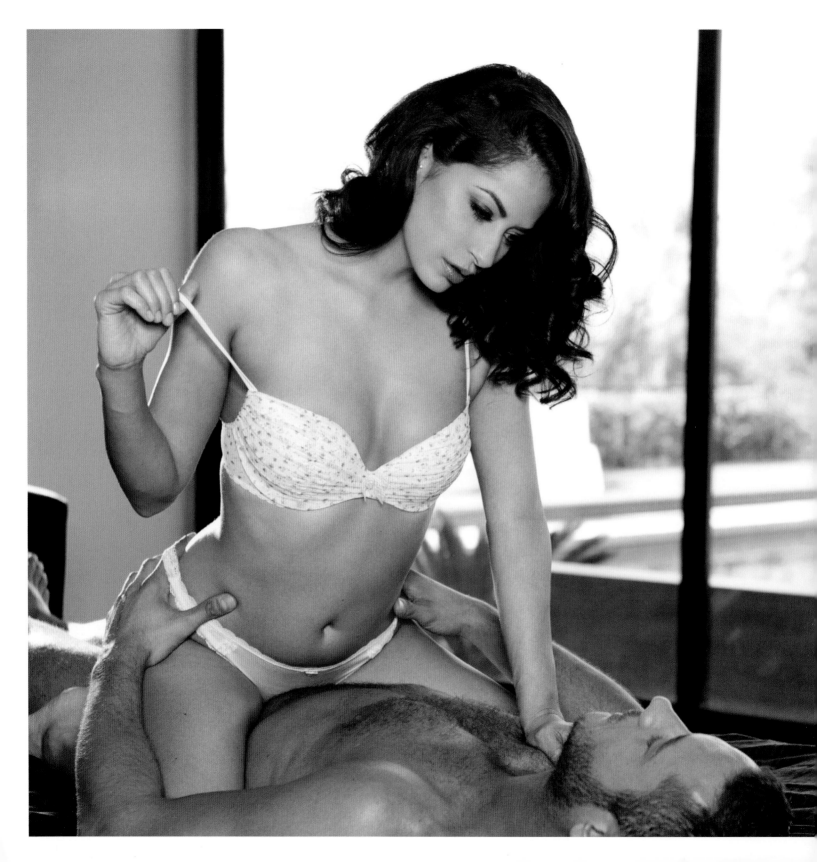

02 ⚀ *Loving Your Sexual Life Span*

If there's one constant thing in life, it's change. Just like your personality, your priorities, your habits, and your body, your sexuality also changes and evolves as time goes by. Your own journey may be different from your peers', and it might differ from your partner's, too. That's a wonderful, natural thing: every woman discovers and explores her sexuality at her own pace, and, through experience, learns what works for her, and when. Sure, there are some norms in terms of hormonal changes and cultural influences—but ultimately, each woman's sexual experience is uniquely her own. In this chapter, I'll show you how to enjoy each step of your sexual life span in your twenties; during and after pregnancy; and in your thirties, forties, fifties, and way beyond.

PUBERTY

But first, let's talk about our very first steps into the world of adult sexuality. That's right: puberty. Does the very thought of those hormone-addled teenage days make you want to run screaming? You're not the only one. Remember how the main character in the film *Carrie* gets her period for the first time in the showers after her swim class in high school? Mortified, Carrie screams for help when she sees the blood, convinced that she's dying. Okay, so it's a bit extreme, but nonetheless, it's a striking example of how education and support—or the lack thereof—can impact the way in which young women view their own bodies during and after puberty.

While it's true that children often do experiment with sexuality during games and play, most initial sexual feelings, thoughts, and physical changes occur during puberty. Puberty—that is, the attainment of sexual maturity—can take place anywhere between the ages of nine and seventeen. During this time, girls experience both physical and emotional changes that impact their interaction with their peers and with the opposite sex. Physically, menstruation begins, breasts start to develop, the clitoris increases in size, body hair begins to sprout under the arms and between the legs, the vulva changes in size and shape, acne is caused by hormone changes, and perspiration increases. In addition to these physical changes, young women also start to experience a variety of new emotions. They may feel embarrassed by their "new" bodies, or they may feel irritable or depressed as a result of the hormonal shifts that instigate puberty. Their thought patterns may change as well, and now is the time when many girls question their self-perception and self-esteem, their identities as young women, and their roles in future relationships with boys and men.

When you went through puberty, you may have reached out to your mother, or another trusted female in your life, for support. If you did, the ways in which she responded to your questions or concerns began to shape your perception of your own body and your budding sexuality—perceptions that affect you to this day. It's important to understand how your experiences during puberty affect your sexuality as an adult. Ask yourself the following questions. Jot down your responses in your journal if you like.

1. Who was the first person you talked to about going through puberty? How did he or she respond? What did that person tell you about those physical changes? Did he or she talk to you about what to expect in terms of emotional changes, or did they come as a surprise?

2. How did you feel about your changing body? Did you feel confident and excited? Did you feel embarrassed or ashamed? How did you cope with those emotions at the time?

3. How has your perception of yourself changed since then? If you could go back in time and give your puberty-age self advice on how to get through this challenging time, what would you tell her?

LOSING IT

It's true: you never forget your first time. Although it sounds a bit clichéd, it's more than likely that your first sexual experience helped shape your long-term attitudes toward sex. You may have had expectations regarding how it would feel, how you'd look while or after doing it, or what your future with your partner might be like. It's possible, though, that your sexual world as a teenager was different from those of many teenagers today. As of 2012, the average age of first sexual penetration was 17.3 for young women living in the United States. Most first experiences happen in exclusive relationships, but those relationships tend to be short-lived. In another 2012 study of girls' virginity loss, researchers found that girls' experiences were nearly all negative: over half of young women who were queried felt strong pressure to have sex for the first time. In a 2003 study, 89% of girls reported feeling pressured by boys to have sex, while 49% of boys reported feeling pressured by girls to have sex. In contrast, 67% of boys felt pressured by other boys, while 53% of girls felt pressured by other girls. Girls, teenagers

reported, perform fellatio on their partners more often than boys perform cunnilingus on theirs. A 2008 study by the Centers for Disease Control and Prevention (CDC) reported that one in four American teenage girls has had an STI. Two-thirds of teenage girls reported wishing that they had waited longer before having sex, and girls who are sexually active are twice as likely to experience teenage depression than their peers who aren't sexually active.

These statistics point toward a worrying pattern that's developed in the sex lives of teenage girls: heavy pressure to "hurry up" and have sex, followed by feelings of guilt and shame after doing it. Once this destructive pattern is set early in a girl's sexual lifestyle, there's nothing to stop it from carrying over into her adult sexual lifestyle—unless she becomes aware of it. And that can take time. Loving yourself as a sexual being is so important. For some of us, it can be a challenging process, and it's okay to want help with that. Visit a supportive sex-positive therapist if you think you might need to discuss negative feelings within a safe environment. That'll help you enjoy your sex life—shame- and guilt-free.

YOUR SEXUAL LIFE SPAN

It's true that each woman experiences her sexuality differently during each stage of her life. That said, there are some norms that lots of women seem to experience. As you age, you might notice shifts in your sex drive, changes in the way your body looks, fluctuations in your self-image, variations in your attitude toward casual sex, and different ideas about what you need from your relationship. Check out this decade-by-decade guide for what to expect.

SEX IN YOUR TWENTIES: IT'S ALL ABOUT SELF-DISCOVERY

Sex in your twenties can be really exciting. You probably haven't been doing it for that long (comparatively), and there are just so many new things—and new men—to try. While Hollywood would have us believe that sex is all dreamy-and-steamy and comes out perfect each time, like some kind of erotic easy-bake cake mix, the fact is, sex is a trial-and-error affair. And now's the time to experiment, whether it's with one partner or with many: that's how you'll learn what turns you on, what doesn't, what you're curious about, and what brings you to orgasm. To get the most out of sex in your twenties, it's essential to:

1. Learn to masturbate. (See chapter 3 for a handy guide to masturbation—no pun intended.) Masturbation is a great way to make yourself feel good, become sexually empowered by taking matters into your own hands—literally—and, ultimately, find out what feels good for you. When you're in touch with your own sexual tastes, and when you know what brings you to orgasm and how you like to get there, you'll really be able to enjoy yourself when you're doing it with your partner.

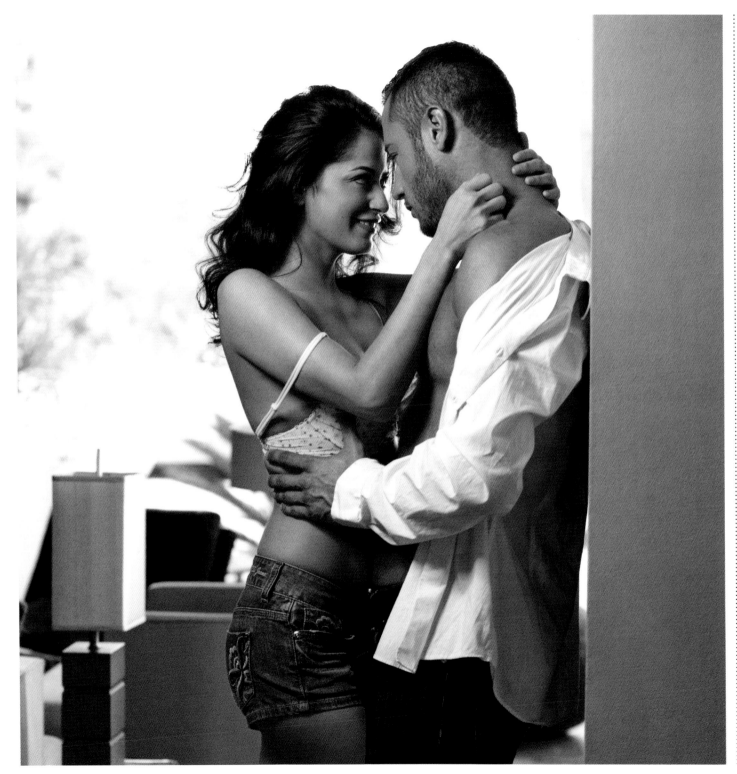

2. *Experiment wisely.* Sexual experimentation in your twenties is both normal and healthy. Maybe you're partying it up at college (when you're not studying, that is); perhaps you're traveling the world, just like you'd always dreamed you'd do; or maybe you've just moved out of your parents' house into your very own place. In your twenties, you're finally free enough to experiment—without knowing that your parents are in the next room, or worrying about gossipy high-school peers finding out about your frolics. Maybe you've started to go out at night and are turning a few heads in your local bars, and you're having casual sex with a couple of guys when you feel like it. Go for it. This is the time to find out what works for you. For some women, casual sex is hot and exciting, while it may feel disconnected and uncomfortable for others. Trust your gut feeling on the subject. And—I can't say it often enough—be sure to use protection if you're having casual sex. Always.

3. *Get tested.* According to a 2011 survey by the CDC, about half of all cases of gonorrhea and chlamydia were diagnosed in people between the ages of twenty and twenty-nine. Since your brain is still developing until you reach your mid-twenties, young men and women of this age may believe that they're untouchable and that their actions won't have negative consequences. Thanks to this kind of "magical thinking," it's all too common for women in their twenties to skip the protection. The result? High rates of STIs (not to mention unexpected pregnancies). Don't let it happen to you. Carry a condom, and if you do have unprotected sex, get tested for STIs right away. Have a frank conversation with your doctor about your birth control options, and always insist on seeing your partner's test results.

PREGNANCY SEX

Pregnancy is a huge milestone in any woman's life: after all, it's the transition period that transforms you into a mother. Lots of women wonder about what'll happen to their sex drive, whether it's safe to have sex during pregnancy, and what changes they'll experience. Again, sexual experiences during pregnancy vary among individuals. Some women report an increase in their sex drives, while others seem to lose interest in sex altogether. Physical discomfort due to symptoms like breast swelling and abdominal cramps may cause some women to avoid physical intimacy. Moodiness and nausea during the first trimester can make newly pregnant women feel not so sexy, and intimacy can be difficult during the last trimester, too, when a larger abdomen and body aches and swelling are at their peak. Then again, some women find sex *more* pleasurable while pregnant. That's because the genitals are the target of increased blood flow during pregnancy, becoming engorged with up to 40% more blood when aroused than they are prepregnancy. Some women also find that their vaginas are more moist during pregnancy, and this natural lubrication can make sex that much more enjoyable.

Naturally, your emotions will also influence the way you feel about sex during pregnancy. It's completely normal to be concerned about the way your body's changing, the progression of the pregnancy, the health of your baby, and what it's like to experience childbirth. You might also be preoccupied with upcoming changes to your work life, your relationship with your partner, or your plans for the future. On top of all this, it's possible that the idea of sex just isn't that sexy.

Talk to your partner about these changes. Your pregnancy affects him, too, of course—not least in the bedroom. Some men find their pregnant partners more attractive than ever before and want sex all the time. Other soon-to-be dads are more apprehensive about sex. They might be afraid of hurting the baby, or they may be

distracted by concerns about fatherhood. That's okay. Work through it together. Tell your partner about the sexual techniques that are safe during pregnancy. Bring him with you to your obstetrician and encourage him to ask questions. Read pregnancy books together to learn the facts. That'll help alleviate his—and your—concerns, and will help you both enjoy pregnancy sex as much as possible.

The good news is that it's perfectly safe to engage in most sexual practices while pregnant. According to gynecologist Dr. Mo Vaziri, "It is important to know that sex is completely safe during pregnancy right up until the water breaks or until the onset of labor. The amniotic sac and the strong muscles of the uterus protect the baby, and the thick mucus plug that seals the cervix helps guard against infection." So feel free to get it on! Oral sex is safe, too (unless your partner has an active herpes outbreak): licking and kissing the vagina is fine, but avoid having your partner blow into your vagina. This can cause an air

embolism, which is a rare but fatal condition. Anal sex, however, is not recommended while pregnant. It could be uncomfortable if you have pregnancy-related hemorrhoids, and it might allow infection-causing bacteria to spread from the rectum to the vagina. If you're in a monogamous relationship, it's no longer necessary to use a condom, since pregnancy isn't a concern anymore (obviously!)—but you should use a condom if you're in an open relationship; if you have sex with a new partner while pregnant; or if you're concerned about a herpes outbreak. During pregnancy, mild cramping after sex can be normal; if the cramping is severe, or lasts more than one to two hours, though, do call your doctor.

Let's move on to the fun part. So, when it comes to pregnancy sex, what's the best way to do it? Lots of sexual positions and techniques are safe and pleasurable during pregnancy, but, regardless of how and where you're doing it, be sure to take it slow and easy and stay aware of your environment (are you on the bed? the floor? in the bath?), your balance (are you comfortable in the position you're in?), and the speed and intensity of his thrusting (is it too fast or too slow?). If you're pregnant, try these positions tonight:

1. Have him lie down on the bed, then straddle him and ease him inside you. This position gives you plenty of control, allowing you to slow down his thrusts, or speed them up.

2. Simply sit him down in a chair and straddle him. It's a hot and spontaneous move—easily and sexily done spur of the moment!

3. Lie down on the bed and get your partner to "spoon" you—and enter you—from behind. His thrusts will be shallower in this position, which will be more comfortable for you as the pregnancy progresses.

4. Sit on the edge of the bed and lean back, supporting yourself with your arms on the bed behind you. Have your partner stand or kneel in front of you, depending on the height of the bed. You can either wrap your legs around your partner, or simply keep them open. This position allows for easy vaginal access, won't place any pressure on your stomach, and lets you support your weight easily.

5. Tell him to enter you from behind, while you're on your knees and elbows on the bed or the floor. (You won't hear him complaining: this position will give him a great view of his penis sliding in and out of you.)

Postpartum Sex
After giving birth, it's possible that sex is the last thing on your mind. You might be completely exhausted, both mentally and physically, due to this massive life change—far too exhausted for sex. Maybe your new schedule as a mom—and a lack of privacy in general, now that there's a newborn around—has made it too challenging to fit regular sex into your routine. Plus, your brain releases oxytocin after giving birth, a hormone that makes you eager to care for and nurture your child. This may mean that you're more likely to want to cuddle than you are to want sex.

That's convenient, actually, since most doctors recommend four to six weeks of abstinence after giving birth so your body has time to heal after delivery. After that, tune in to how you feel—physically and emotionally. Some women feel ready for sex sooner rather than later, while others aren't ready for months. Take your time. The reality is that your body has just experienced a physical trauma and it needs to heal. When you do decide to have sex again, it can help to:

Try positions in which thrusting is more shallow, like the spooning position recommended earlier. Or get on top of him so you can control the depth of penetration. Try the L-shape position, which lets you both relax and take your time: get your partner to lie on his side. You lie down so that your body is perpendicular to his, with your legs over his hips. It's easy to stimulate your clitoris in this position, too.

Go slow, and be gentle with yourself. Don't expect to race right back into fast, intensely passionate prepregnancy sex. Do it slow and steamy instead of hot and fast; slower sex might even give you both stronger orgasms.

Talk to your partner. Be honest about how you're feeling—and get him to do the same. Let him reassure you that it's okay to rediscover sex at your own pace.

"Sex after the first baby was fine, because I had a C-section. Since the second baby, which was a vaginal birth, it has been almost nonexistent. First, it was because it was too dry and painful. That lasted for eight months, because I breast-fed and I didn't make enough estrogen to fully heal my vagina. I've taken two rounds of estrogen cream, and I'm on my third. I would have to stop breast-feeding in order for my hormone levels to go back to normal, but that's not an option. Since my vaginal birth I do not allow hubby to give me oral pleasure, which was a HUGE part of our sex life. It's because I don't feel the same there: I think about how a baby went through there, and it grosses me out." —Shirley, 33

You may have just given birth, but that doesn't mean you can't get pregnant again right away. So make sure you've thought about birth control. (Even if you're breast-feeding, you're still able to get pregnant.) Birth control pills that contain estrogen and progesterone may cause blood clots after giving birth, so do consult your doctor about which birth control will work best for you. Think about using condoms: they're an easy and nonhormonal way to prevent getting pregnant again so soon after your recent delivery.

Intimacy After Pregnancy
It's almost impossible to find time to do *anything* with a newborn around. Doing the laundry? Washing your hair? Peeing? All things of the past. Nonetheless, it's still possible to squeeze a little much-needed intimacy into the early days of new motherhood.

Nap time for the little one means one-on-one time for you and your partner. You might be exhausted, but do use this precious time to connect with each other—even if briefly. Touch, hold, and kiss each other as much as possible. Try an afternoon quickie (after you're healed, of course), or indulge in a passionate makeout session.

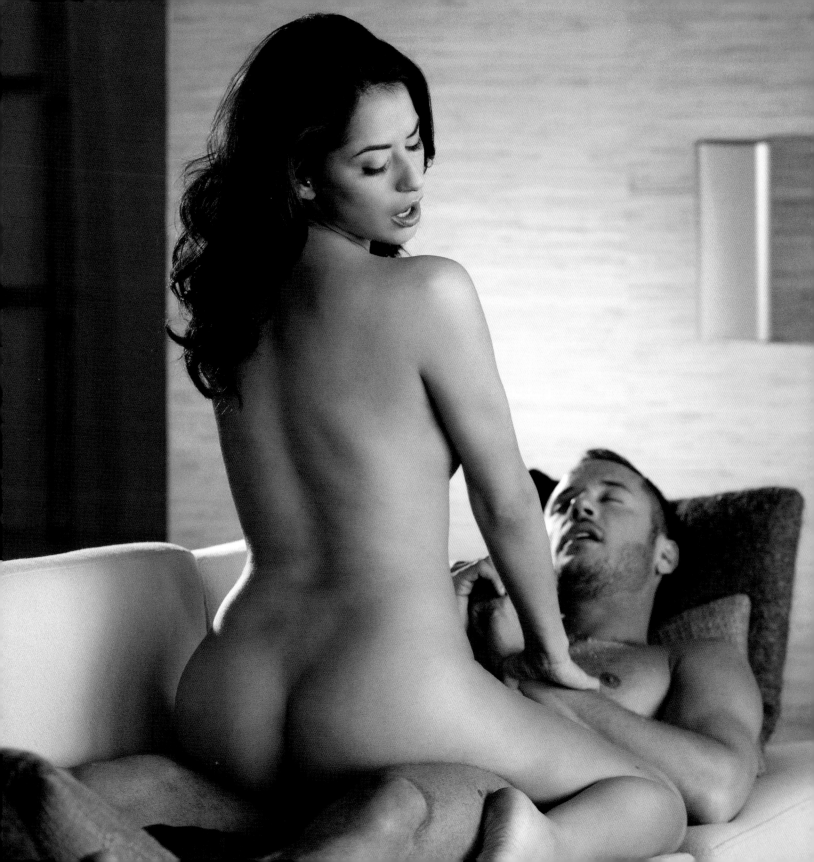

Take your body for a test run. It takes time to get used to the changes in your body and the new sensations that pregnancy, delivery, and new motherhood have brought with them. Spend some time alone while your baby is sleeping and explore yourself. Start by caressing your body, paying attention to the new shapes of your hips, breasts, and stomach. That'll help you get used to these changes. They're yours—and they're beautiful. Go ahead and accept them.

Use a hand mirror and masturbate. Getting used to your bodily changes will help you feel more comfortable being sexual with your partner. The first time you try, start by gently massaging the outer parts of your vulva. Use the mirror to notice the ways in which your body has changed after birth. Your vulva might have changed in color, shape, and its amount of natural lubrication. If you're using your fingers only, feel free to use a water-based lubricant to add moisture, since it can be absorbed into the body naturally. Slip a finger inside and notice how your vagina feels. If you had a vaginal delivery, it might not feel as tight as it did prebirth, but don't worry: the vagina is very elastic, and its tightness can be regained with time and by doing Kegel exercises to strengthen the pelvic floor muscles. You may be in for a pleasant surprise, too. Many women report that they are *more* orgasmic postbirth, possibly due to the increased blood flow to the pelvic area.

SEX IN YOUR THIRTIES: WELCOME TO THE DIRTY THIRTIES

Thanks to the media and so-called women's magazines, you might have heard that women reach their sexual peak in their thirties—and that they should be having the most mind-blowing sex of their lives at this stage, because it's either now or never. That's a lot of pressure—and it's simply not true. Dr. Ruth Westheimer, the well-known sex expert who is now in her eighties, believes that each woman's sexuality has many peaks over her sexual life span, and that these peaks vary from woman to woman.

At this point in your life, you may notice changes in your body. Some women have had children, which may have impacted their body shape. Whether or not you're a mom, you might have gained weight, seen a few gray hairs. Maybe your breasts have begun to droop a bit. Your metabolism may have slowed since your twenties, and your testosterone—the hormone that drives sexual desire, even in women—might have started to taper. In addition to these physical changes, your sexual availability may also have changed.

The challenges of a demanding career, devoting time to your relationship, or your role as a mother—to name just a few of the life challenges that lots of us face—may mean that you've got less time to be spontaneous and experimental. Perhaps sex has become planned: instead of doing it spur of the moment, you save it for Sunday mornings. You love your kids, but maybe having them crawl into bed with you at night is a passion-killer. That's all completely normal—but that doesn't mean it's not frustrating.

That said, there are so many great things about sex in your thirties. Your twenties were all about trial and error. You learned plenty about what *doesn't* work for you. By now, you might be enjoying a calmer, committed relationship. Your inhibitions have decreased while your self-esteem, self-knowledge, and sexual confidence have increased. It's a great place to be. Here's how to get the most out of sex in your thirties:

1. *Make the time.* Maybe you're single and career-focused, working eight days a week—or maybe you're a full-time mother of four. (Or both.) Regardless, you do need to make time for sex. It's okay to plan a little. Talk to your partner, and agree on a time for regular romps—and how frequent you want those romps to be. Then hold each other to it (literally and figuratively). If you have kids, plan an adults-only evening so that you can focus on each other. Or consider making a new rule for your kids: make it clear to them that there are appropriate times for them to enter your bedroom or other personal space.

2. *Set boundaries.* During your sexually active twenties, you learned a lot about yourself. Now, you're very firm on how you expect to be treated in relationships—and in the bedroom. Trust your gut instincts. If you feel like something's not right in a relationship, take a step back for a moment. Ask yourself why you might be experiencing these feelings—then do something about it. Set boundaries with your sexual expectations, and make sure the men in your life respect them. This is *your* time to get what you want.

3. *Stay active.* Your thirties may be the first decade in which you notice a significant decrease in your metabolism. Maybe you're eating the same way you have for years—but suddenly, you're struggling with weight gain. Now's the time to develop new habits. Lock down a regular workout routine and stick to it, come the proverbial hell or high water. Eat healthfully (but do allow yourself a treat from time to time). A healthy diet and exercise plan increase your energy—and that translates to sexual energy. Staying in good shape also helps you enjoy sex: you'll be able to engage in more positions, you'll have better kinesthetic awareness, and you'll like the way you look while doing it. All this will help you down the line, too. The experiences of aging and menopause are more comfortable when you've got less body fat, increased bone density, and less stress.

4. *Accept yourself after the baby.* If you're a new mom, it's important to know that it's normal to feel less sexual and more—well, tired. (After all, you've just created a human.) Plus, after birth, your body releases hormones that increase the

"I feel like my sex drive is stronger than ever. Instead of giving to partners that are poor choices, or feeling shame with casual sex, I choose to engage only in the sexual behaviors that match what I know I feel good about."
—Nicolette, 32

desire to bond and decrease the desire for sex. It takes time and energy to cope with these immense physical, psychological, and life changes. Be good to yourself, and accept yourself for the person you are at the moment.

5. Manage stress healthfully. Stress does take a toll on both your body and your sexuality. In your twenties, it might've been easy to power through this stress despite late nights and less sleep—but in your thirties, your body will have its revenge, if you're not careful. High stress levels produce cortisol, which reduces testosterone, the sex drive hormone. The best way to counteract that? Have sex! It reduces stress. It's also important to exercise regularly, see a therapist to learn personalized stress management tools (if necessary), and get enough sleep (ideally, seven to nine hours per night).

SEX IN YOUR FORTIES: KNOWING YOUR SEXUAL SELF

As you move into your forties, you'll have become stronger and more experienced as a woman. Age does bring a few new challenges with it, though. On average, women begin to enter perimenopause in their early forties. This term refers to the changes that take place in your body prior to menopause, and one of the symptoms is the fluctuation of estrogen levels. This can have a huge impact on your sexual self, since it can cause thinning of the vaginal walls as well as a reduction in your body's natural lubrication. That can make sex undesirable and uncomfortable; in some instances, penetration can cause trauma and even injury. If you're experiencing dryness, try using lubricants. (There are a variety of water- and silicone-based lubricants on the market. Check out my guide on page 171 to figure out which ones might work best for you.) Consult your gynecologist about vaginal wall thinness. He or she may be able to prescribe a cream to help thickness. Also, the muscles of the pelvic floor start to weaken with age. That can cause a decrease in sensation in the vaginal area, may make it harder to retain urine, and can even cause vaginal prolapse. Keep your pelvic muscles strong by doing Kegel exercises. (Kegels are easy: see #2 in the following list for a quick rundown on how to do them.)

Of course, men feel the effects of aging, too. You might notice that it's harder for your partner to achieve an erection, or that the erection itself may not be as hard. That doesn't need to stop you. Remember, sex doesn't need to revolve around a penis and its erection. (Plus, a man doesn't need a fully erect penis to achieve a satisfying orgasm.) However, if erectile problems seem to be chronic, or if they're causing him distress, encourage your partner to consult his doctor to discuss his options, such as erectile dysfunction medication.

It's not all doom and gloom, though. Sex in your forties can be incredibly exciting and rewarding. Whether you've been committed to a single partner for some time or had a number of relationships, you've learned a great deal about your sexuality, your body, and what works well for you. Be proud of being strong, and of

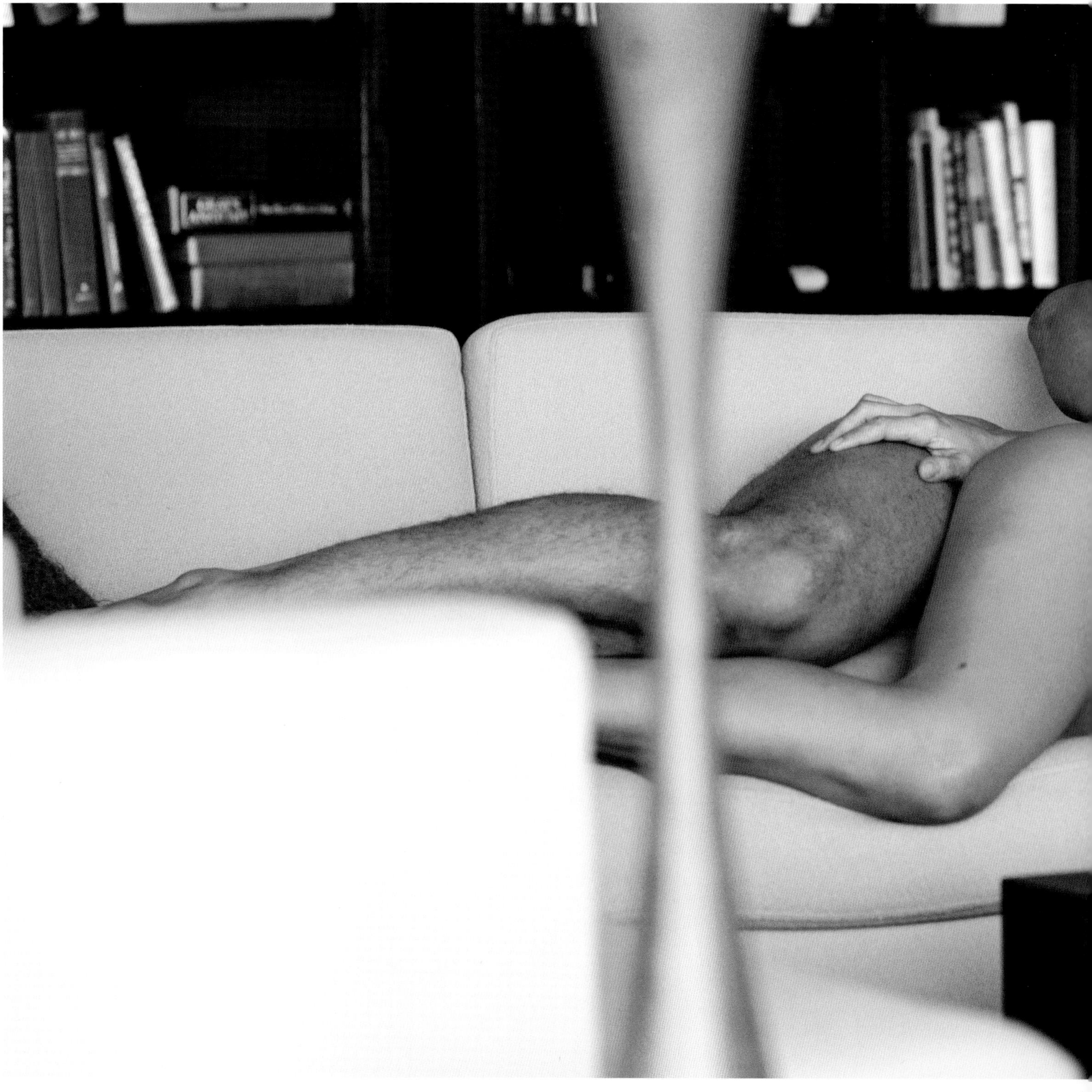

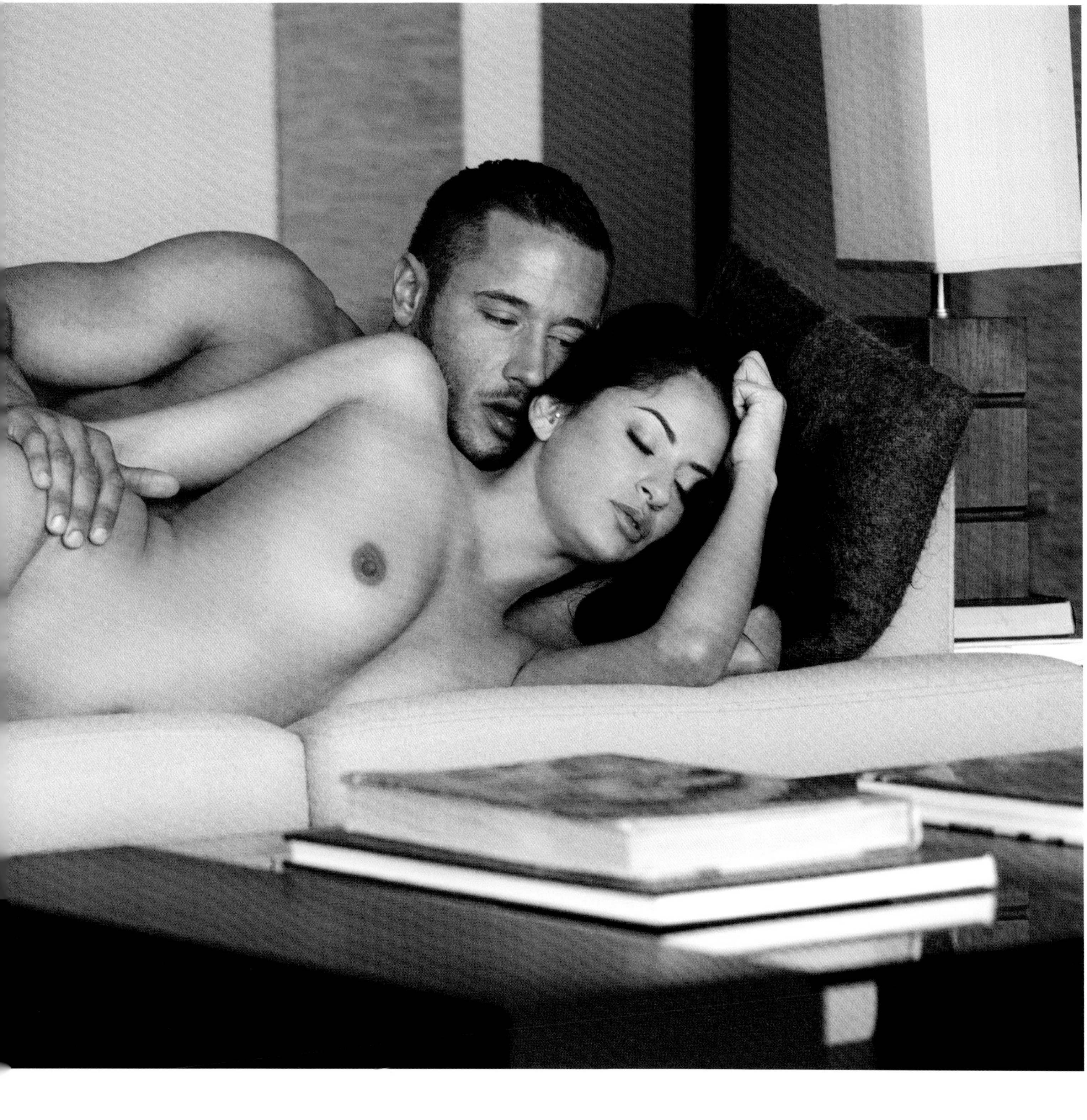

being on such intimate terms with your sexual self. Women in their forties often tell me that they remember how beautiful they were when they were younger, and they regret not having appreciated their own beauty to its fullest. Regardless of your age, though, it's vital to stay in the here and how. Admire yourself. Notice how beautiful your body is right now, and acknowledge what you love about it.

Here's how to enjoy sex throughout your forties:

1. Reach for the lube. Vaginal dryness can happen to women of any age, but it often becomes an issue in your forties due to the change in estrogen production as you age. It's not that you're not turned on enough: your natural lubrication might not match your level of arousal. It's easy to get frustrated with the lube choices available to you at the drugstore—most of them are water-based, and end up being sticky, goopy messes. They also include a preservative that may cause irritation. Silicone lubricants are much more slippery and they last a long time but are generally more expensive. If you're prone to yeast infections or urinary tract infections, try hybrid or glycerin-free lubes.

2. Tighten it up with Kegels. Not only do Kegel exercises tighten up the vaginal muscles, which makes for sex that feels tighter, but they also help to generally strengthen the muscles of the pelvic floor, which holds and supports all of your reproductive organs. When your pelvic floor is tight, you'll orgasm more easily, you'll enjoy more controlled vaginal sex, you'll notice a reduction in urinary incontinence, and you'll prevent vaginal and uterine prolapse. Kegel exercises are easy. To start, try to stop your urine stream midflow and notice how it feels. Later—when you're not urinating, of course!—position yourself comfortably in front of a mirror and repeat that movement. You should be able to see your perineum—the space between your vagina and anus—contract. Your goal is to hold the contraction for 10 seconds, and repeat about 5 times. But if you're new to Kegels, start with contractions of just 2-3 seconds and build up to 10 seconds over time. Do this two or three times per day.

3. Check in with your gynecologist. At your yearly checkup, ask your doctor to test your hormone levels. This will tell you whether you're entering perimenopause. It's important to know so you can make better, safer choices for your body. Also, you want to check in with your doctor about updating your birth control. The diaphram that you used in your twenties and thirties may not fit your changing body, for example. Or perhaps your relationship status has changed from a monogamous relationship to openly dating due to divorce. If so, you'll need a birth control method that also protects against STIs.

4. Don't get lazy with birth control. Hormone levels fluctuate a lot in the forties due to perimenopause. You may even notice that you occasionally skip your menstrual cycle or that your cycle becomes lighter. It is easy to get complacent with birth control or mistakenly think that your body is "done" with pregnancy—particularly if you had your children in your twenties and thirties and aren't actively trying to conceive. However, pregnancy can happen in your forties, so you want to talk to your doctor about the right birth control method for you—and use it. Every single time.

"For the first time, I was so dry that I needed to buy a lubricant. Shopping at the local drugstore was embarrassing and confusing. I found websites like Babeland.com that had information on different lubricants. After using the right kind, my sex and intimacy has drastically improved." —Arlene, 56

5. Put your relationship first. Make your relationship with your partner a priority—even over your children. It'll have a positive effect on your kids: it shows them that they're in a safe, stable environment. Plus, modeling a loving and healthy relationship for your children will help them make positive choices when they form their own relationships later in life. Prioritizing your relationship also lets you enjoy one-on-one time with your partner without feeling guilty for not spending that time with your kids or as a family.

6. Have sex once a week (even if you don't feel like it). The fact is, life gets in the way, sex drives decrease, and sometimes you might feel you've settled into a lifestyle pattern that doesn't include sex. That can make you and your partner feel disconnected from one another. But that's a pattern you can change. Just as your sexual feelings can cause you to behave sexually, the opposite is also true: sexual behaviors will result in sexual feelings. So "make" yourself have sex once a week. You might not be in the mood for it at first, but you'll get more aroused right after you start. Honestly. And afterward—in addition to being sexually satisfied!—you'll feel a deeper, stronger connection with your partner.

SEX IN YOUR FIFTIES: IT'S ALL ABOUT PLEASURE

For most of your adult sexual life, you've probably been focused on one of two things: getting pregnant, or *not* getting pregnant. By the time you reach your fifties, that's changed. You may be married, in a committed relationship, or newly dating (close to 20% of members of dating websites are over fifty). If you've reached menopause, your chances of getting pregnant are virtually nonexistent. However—and this is a *big* however—unless you haven't had your period for a full year, you're still in perimenopause, and therefore, you are still able to get pregnant. That comes as surprising news to a lot of women—but it's absolutely true. And aside from pregnancy, you're still at risk for sexually transmitted diseases. With divorce rates in the United States hovering around 50%, men and women who haven't been single in decades are joining the dating pool, and some of them are treating casual and "dating" sex like sex within their marriages—that is, they're not using protection. The result? The rate of STIs among people over fifty has more than doubled in the past decade.

"Sex in your sixties/seventies/eighties: postmenopausal changes can be hormonal, physiological, and anatomical. Pelvic organ prolapse becomes more prevalent with age, especially if a woman has had prior vaginal births and may require surgical repair. Regular Kegel exercises can help minimize the severity of prolapse. Decreased estrogen and testosterone levels can cause the problems mentioned above and decrease libido significantly. Vaginal creams, lubricants, and hormone therapy can help alleviate some of these issues." –Mo Vaziri, M.D., F.A.C.O.G.

I'm not trying to scare you, though. There's a simple solution. Just ask your doctor about the best form of birth control for your lifestyle, and always use condoms. And be open with your partner. If he's in your age range, it's likely that he's dealing with the changes that aging brings to his own sexuality. And enjoy yourself. This is the first decade in which sex is just about the two of you, with no other agenda. Focus on foreplay, touch, connection, and sensation instead of racing to orgasm. Here are some ways to get the most out of sex in your fifties:

1. Dating? Use a condom. Learn where to buy condoms and how to put them on (see my easy guide on page 27). Carry them with you if sex is a possibility. It's never too late to learn how to protect yourself.

2. Slow it down. When it comes to getting it on, both men and women in their fifties may need additional time to warm up. So treat foreplay as part of the main course, rather than an appetizer you need to hurry through to get to penetration. Try kicking things off with an erotic massage session—or spend time getting to know each other's erogenous zones inside and out. There are so many ways to make love aside from vaginal penetration—and they can make sex more intimate, not less. This is the time to have sex purely for pleasure and connection, so take your time and enjoy it.

3. Choose your self-perception. In your fifties, you might have reached a crossroads in terms of how you perceive your own sexuality. After menopause, some women choose to think negatively about themselves, their body, and their sexuality. They choose to "give up," so to speak, and to accept a life without intimate or sexual connection. Others choose to embrace their own sexual expression, and enjoy a growing sense of self-worth. (After all, you're finally rid of periods, PMS, and pregnancy worries.) Some women in their fifties have told me they're having the best sex of their lives.

SEX IN YOUR SIXTIES: HOT AND HEALTHY SEX

The Golden Girls TV show proved to us that sex in your sixties is not only possible, but it can also be very satisfying and lots of fun. In fact, it can be better than ever. And what's more, it's good for you. Sex increases the blood flow to the genitals, promoting blood circulation to the genital tissue and to the entire body. Doing it, though, may require some planning now: it might not be possible to be as spontaneous or uninhibited as you were when you were younger. That means that sex may be less frequent—but it can be more connective and intimate. When you have sex, stay in the present and enjoy each moment. Try not to take sex and pleasure for granted. At any age, sex is an amazing gift. You may have health concerns or insecurities about your body—but it's likely that your partner does, too. About half of American couples in their sixties report that they are sexually active, and those who are report greater satisfaction with their relationships. The moral of the story is, the more sex you have, the happier you'll be with your relationship.

It's important to keep an eye on your health, though. At this age, you or your partner might be on medication or have had other health concerns. Injuries; health problems such as diabetes, high blood pressure, and heart conditions; and medications can all impact sex drive, so talk to your doctor about how these factors could impact your sex life. Here's how to get the most out of sex in your sixties:

1. Just do it. Adopt a now-or-never attitude with everything from fashion and hobbies to sex. If you're not trying lots of new things, ask yourself why. Now is the time to experiment and enjoy yourself, both in and out of the bedroom.

2. Plan the passion. Planning your intimacy can be more sexy, not less. Since lubricants and a relaxing setting can really help both you and your partner to become aroused, choose a time and place for sex so you can set the mood and enjoy each other without interruption.

3. Adjust your expectations. As you age, there'll be changes in your sexuality and the way you express it—and those changes will be individual to you. Change your sexual expectations to remove the pressure of penetration and ejaculation: after all, there's more than just one way to do it! And sexuality and sensuality can be enjoyed without necessarily reaching orgasm.

4. Love the body you have. The reality is, your body has changed. Embrace it and love it for what it has done for you. You're still very much in control of your own body, and healthy eating and exercise can do wonders for your sex life. Increase your muscle strength by doing weight-bearing exercise, like brisk walking, yoga, and dancing. You can feel sexier by treating yourself to flattering lingerie, tinted lotions, or spray tans, or surrounding yourself with soft, glowing lighting.

"When my husband became impotent due to a stroke, it was a very difficult time for him because he did not want to lose his ability to have sexual relations. I needed to assure him that he was loved and wanted and would be taken care of for the rest of our lives whether he was sexual or not. He eventually understood this and we became the closest of friends. We were more than lovers; we were inseparable." –Barbara, 72

SEX IN YOUR SEVENTIES: ACCEPTANCE AND SELF-SOOTHING

When you're in your seventies, your sexual priorities will probably have changed. Pain from years of a postmenopausal lack of estrogen may make vaginal penetration difficult, while pain and discomfort from health issues such as arthritis, shingles, or mastectomies may make getting close less comfortable. And since women typically live longer than men, some women find themselves alone after long marriages, and they have no desire to search for a new partner. Some women don't miss sex; their sex drives may have decreased, and they aren't bothered if they're not getting any—although it can be difficult to deal with society's pressure on women to be sexual at every age. Other women in their seventies, however, are still very interested in sex. At seventy-one, Jane Fonda said that she "doesn't feel so good because she is in pain. But, I am happier, the sex is better, and I understand life better. I don't want to be young again." A ringing endorsement for sex in your

seventies! About a quarter of married couples in this age bracket are still sexually active—but even if you're not having sex, you don't need to sacrifice intimacy and pleasure. Sex doesn't have to be about "getting off": it can be about self-pleasure and self-love, too.

Here are some ways to get the most out of sex and sexuality in your seventies and beyond:

1. Masturbate. Like sex, masturbation doesn't need to be orgasm-oriented. Love your body through self-massage and by touching and caressing your vagina. Love yourself with the same care you'd expect from a partner.

2. Accept yourself, moment by moment. It's okay to be hot and ready for sex—or to be completely unconcerned with it. Go with your instincts. If you experience pain and discomfort during sex, take it slow, or change your technique. Listen to your body and your emotions, and let them be your guide.

3. *Let go of cultural pressures.* Western culture puts pressure on women to be sexual, when sometimes we simply aren't. Sometimes we're tigresses—but there are times when we just don't feel like sexual animals. Either way, pay no attention to cultural and media messages that encourage you to be something you're not. Say no to guilt and shame. Love your body and your life experiences—both inside the bedroom and out of it.

As women, we've all got lots in common when it comes to our sexual life spans, like puberty, adulthood, the possibility of pregnancy, the upswings and downswings of sex drive, menopause, and aging. No matter what age you are, though, sex at its best can be about self-discovery, self-pleasure, connectivity, and self-acceptance. Each woman's body, circumstances, and desires are different, and the most important thing is that we love ourselves at every stage of our lives. Read on to find out how to boost your sexual self-esteem in a big way.

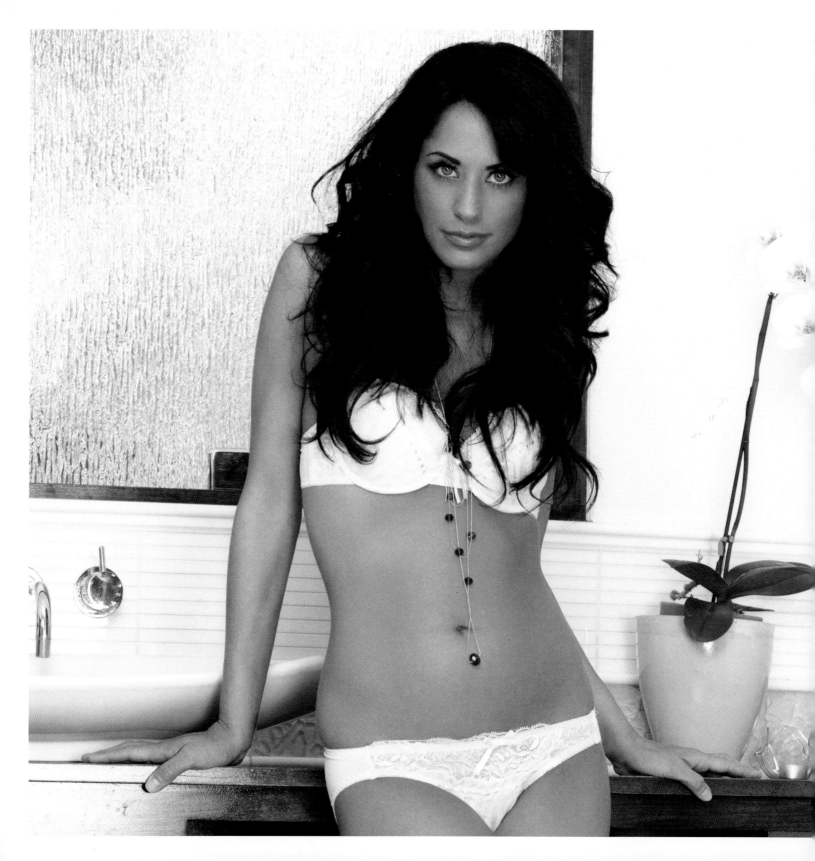

03 *Boosting Your Sexual Self-Esteem*

When you were a little girl, you probably didn't judge yourself when it came to your body. As you aged, comments by and reactions from your parents, peers, friends, partners, and even the media may have started to shape your views on your own body and your sexuality. Overhearing someone calling a woman who dressed in an overtly sexual manner "slutty," being on the receiving end of a shame-inducing comment, or noticing a negative physical reaction to another woman's body can have a huge impact on how you think, feel, and, ultimately, act in your adult sexual life.

And it can lead you to associate shame, guilt, and self-loathing with sexuality. Conversely, though, the greater your sexual self-esteem, the more confidence you'll have in yourself, your sexual behavior, and your identity as a sexual woman. Sexual self-esteem has to be built and cultivated—and this chapter will show you how to do just that. I'll show you how to figure out your sexual priorities and give you a crash course in masturbation. Plus, I'll clue you in on how to set sexual boundaries with your partner, and—most important—help you respect, admire, and enjoy your own body.

SO WHAT IS SEXUAL SELF-ESTEEM—AND HOW DO YOU GET IT?

Sexual self-esteem is, simply, the way you view yourself as a sexual being. Just like your nonsexual self-esteem can determine patterns of thought, emotion, and action, so can your sexual self-esteem. It's not just how adept you are at mastering a complicated sex act or how many men you've slept with. Sexual self-esteem is far more holistic, and includes the way you view your body, your sexual anatomy, and your relationship choices. While positive, pleasurable sex can improve your sexual self-esteem, sex that's not in tune with your core beliefs can actually lower your sexual self-esteem. For instance, if a woman enjoys sex primarily within committed relationships and the securities that come with them, she'll be able to build her sexual self-esteem when she receives the emotional feedback that comes with that type of sex: knowing that her partner is affectionate and reliable, being able to communicate openly, and looking forward to long-term commitment. That's because she's making choices that match her personal code of values.

But if that same woman chooses one-night stands and casual sex, she'll experience cognitive dissonance, because the needs that correspond to her personal values aren't being met. Cognitive dissonance can cause psychological distress and lower your sexual self-esteem—which, in turn, can lead you to engage in even riskier behaviors. This vicious cycle not only creates poor sexual self-esteem, but it can also lead to serious mental health issues. That's why it's vital to take an active role in educating yourself about your sexuality. It's also important to make time for a little self-reflection in order to become aware of both your strengths and your tender points. After all, no matter how sexually confident you think you are, there's always more to learn about yourself, your sexuality, and your relationships.

SEXUAL SELF-ESTEEM STARTS BY SEARCHING WITHIN

Proactive choices are key when it comes to sexual self-esteem. Since it's determined by your daily actions, observations, and psychological outlook, taking positive steps toward tuning in to your sexual self-esteem is essential. Congratulations: by buying this book, you've already done just that! Now keep going. Improve your sexual self-esteem by taking a moment to ask yourself these questions:

1. Do you use sex as a means of improving your self-worth or manipulating your partners?

2. Do you find yourself sexually valuable only when receiving validation—such as compliments—from others?

3. Do you ever feel regretful about your sexual experiences?

4. Are you uncomfortable with the numbers of partners that you've had?

5. Do you feel you need to drink alcohol in order to be intimate?

6. Are you hyper-aware of how you position your body during sex, for fear that it might look unattractive or unflattering?

7. Have you faked an orgasm to avoid feeling awkward?

If you answered yes to any of these questions, you may need to take a good look at what motivates you to engage in less-than-healthy sex. Relying on sex for self-worth and validation actually diminishes the intimacy and connection that comes with sex because it prevents you from focusing on the act itself. If you're experiencing regret in connection with some of your sexual experiences, you may be participating in sex that isn't aligned with your core beliefs. For example, if you're happiest having connective sex with a single partner but continue to engage in one-night stands, you'll begin to view sex as an act that inspires regret, not pleasure. Of course, that works the other way around, too: if you enjoy casual sex, you might feel trapped or tied down by sex within the confines of a relationship. Your sexual beliefs are up to you.

Remember, as long as you're a consenting adult and engaging in sexually safe behavior, there is no such thing as "wrong" sex. Use the information in this chapter as a guideline, and enjoy discovering what works best for you.

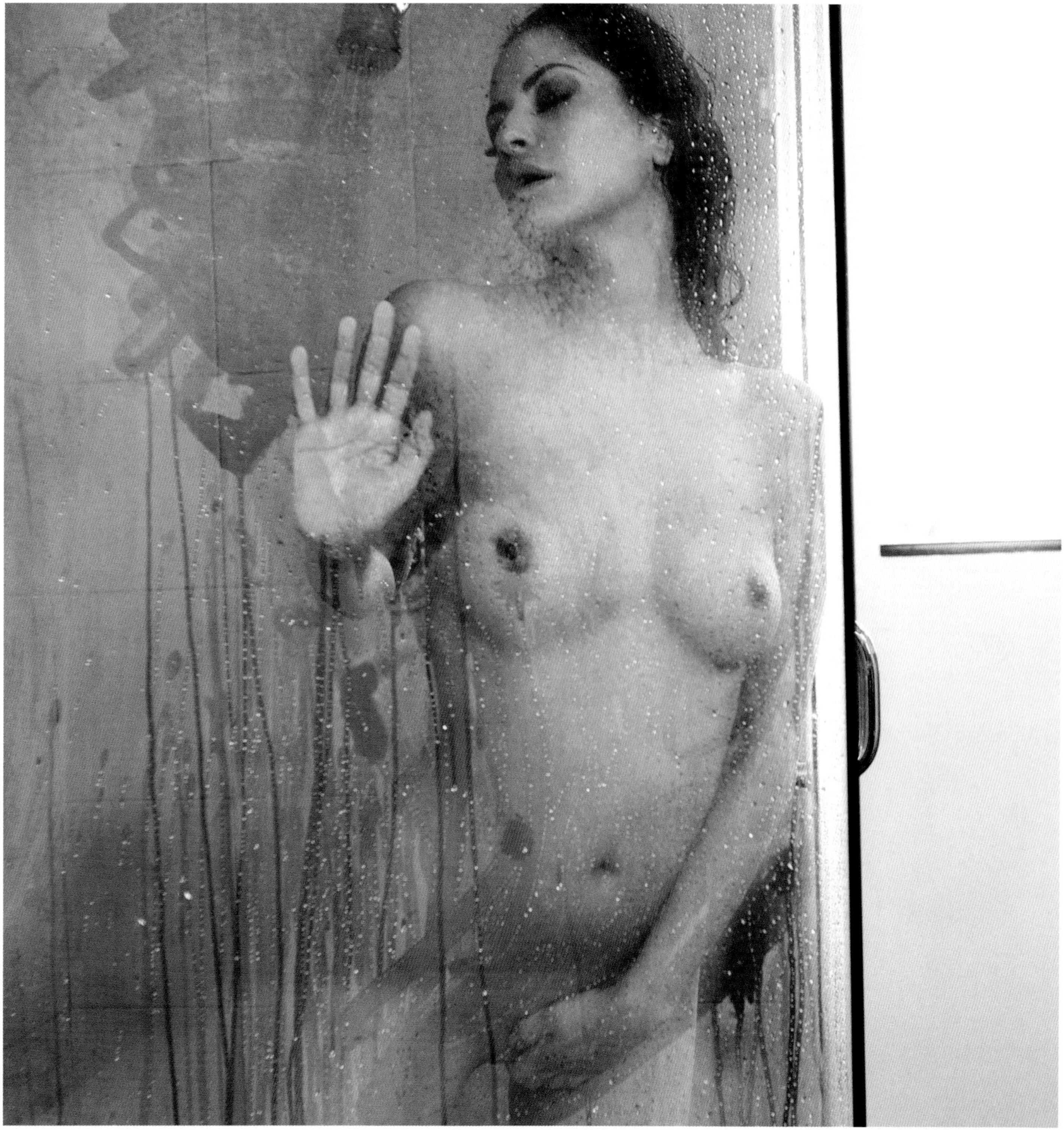

Get out your favorite journal or notebook and settle down in a comfortable, relaxed environment. What was the best sexual experience of your life? What about the worst? Write about each using as much detail as possible. Who was your partner? Where did it happen? Were you sober, or had you been drinking or using other mind-altering substances? How satisfying was it? Can you remember your thoughts before, during, and after each experience? What are your lasting impressions of these encounters—the ones that have stayed with you to this day? Now, think about what made each experience positive or negative. This will help you learn what to include in your future sexual encounters—and what to avoid. Both are important: the things that work for you and the things that don't comprise your core sexual values.

You might find that you feel shaky about some aspects of sexual confidence, such as the way you perceive your appearance, your sexual skills, your perception of your sexual self, the way you compare yourself to others, or how you experience shame or guilt in connection with your sexuality. That's okay. Everyone has sexual strengths and weaknesses. Sometimes our confidence runs dry because our bodies have been shamed, or because we focus on comparing our bodies with other women's. If you lack confidence in your appearance in general, or if you dislike the way your body looks during sex, here are some ways to make yourself more body-confident:

1. Exercise. I can't say it enough: exercise reduces stress, boosts your mood, and, just as important, helps you know and love your body. Sign up for classes such as pole-dancing or belly-dancing, which are specifically focused on the movement of the female body. Whatever you choose, pick a form of exercise you like, and do it regularly. Choosing to exercise can be a huge boost to your overall self-esteem and confidence, because you're actively supporting your body in a positive, healthy way.

2. Stop comparing. Quit comparing your body to other women's—especially celebrities and other women in the media spotlight. Look at the women around you, and notice what real women look like. Start to love yourself by getting to know your body and by focusing on treating it healthfully and well. Or browse real-women websites instead, like mybodygallery.com and theshapeofamother.com, which are dedicated to posting images of so-called average women instead of the very small pocket of women who appear in the media: those women are real women too, but they represent a tiny, tiny percentage of the population.

3. Look for what you like. Rather than being negative and self-critical, take a moment to compliment yourself on what you like about your body. Instead of focusing on the cellulite on the back of your thighs, focus on how shapely your legs are. Dwell on that for a while. The next time you find yourself beset by negative body thoughts—and it happens to all of us—call that compliment to mind and admire yourself all over again.

4. Pick a goddess. Identify several women who embody your ideals of strength and sexuality. They could be women you know in your own life, or well-known women like sportswomen, politicians, activists, or artists. Getting inspired by these real-life goddesses can be really motivational—and they can also act as symbols for the diverse forms that female beauty takes.

5. Be the change. Women's bodies should be praised, not shamed. So, as Gandhi said, be the change you wish to see in the world. Give other women compliments on their figures, and mean it. Avoid slut shaming. By "slut shaming," I mean the act of being negatively critical of other women's sexual identities. Don't put other women down for how sexual—or nonsexual— they may look or act. Your sexuality is your own, to use as you please, and so is hers.

BOOST YOUR SEXUAL IQ

Maybe you're unsure about your sexual skills. If so, you can be confident that they'll be up to speed if you take the time and effort to brush up on your knowledge and skills. Unfortunately, our bodies, and our partners, don't come with an owner's manual on how to have great sex. You may have had sex education in junior high, but most sexual information (unless you were lucky enough to be in a very progressive environment) revolves around the basic mechanics of intercourse and pregnancy prevention. The fact is, most people get more education in how to drive a car than they do on how to have healthy and fulfilling sex. And not unlike driving a car, there is no substitute for actual experience, but you need to have some knowledge before you get behind the wheel so the experience is fun and safe.

Read a book about sex. (Like this one!) Reading about sexual skills is a fun way to teach yourself new things, and to be reassured about what's "normal." Another strategy is to watch good porn or read erotica. Watching people have sex is a great way to learn new techniques and feel confident in the skills that you have. (It might turn you on, too.) But when it comes to porn, it's important to choose wisely. Some types of porn deliver unrealistic, sanitized versions of sex or show acts that are just plain unsafe—and that isn't something you want to learn. Look for porn that's directed by women, or that's produced by conscientious companies that depict women and their bodies in a positive way. And check out the Sinclair Institute's Better Sex video series (www.sinclairinstitute.com). Their respectful, "real-life" sex education videos show sex as it really is.

Another great way to learn about sex is to take a class at your local sex-toy boutique. Lots of sex-toy shops offer how-to events or workshops, so you can learn from the experts in a safe, relaxed environment. It's a fun way to get information, ask questions, and listen to the questions of others. Or visit websites like babeland.com and check out their video tutorials. Then practice your new hand-job or blow-job techniques on a dildo. You might have already seen it done in class—now try it at home. Seriously! It'll help you get a feel for things, so to speak. Watch yourself in the mirror while you're doing it so you can see how hot it'll look from your partner's angle. Most important, ask for feedback. That'll help reassure you that you're already doing a great job. Ask your partner to tell you, explicitly, which sex acts he thinks you're best at. Be sure to set the parameter that this is positive feedback only. You want to hear what you are good at so you can boost your confidence and expand on that skill set.

MASTURBATION: LOVE YOURSELF

Masturbation is a healthy, positive, and empowering act, and most women have tried it: in fact, studies have shown that between 60% and 70% of women masturbate. Not that you'll hear most women talk about it. Due to the stigmas attached to women's sexuality, and the cultural assumption that people in general—and women in particular—shouldn't talk about sex, it's likely that even more women masturbate: they're just not comfortable with admitting it. And it makes sense that so many women do it. One of the biggest benefits of masturbation is, simply, that it feels good. Touching yourself and bringing yourself to orgasm is pleasurable, and being aware of this is empowering and satisfying. It can also improve your sexual relationships: by masturbating, you're discovering what feels good, and that'll help you get the most out of sex with your partner. Psychologically, many mental health circles agree that masturbation can reduce depression and increase self-esteem.

So why doesn't anyone tell you how to do it? You probably had sex education in school, and your parents might have given you the standard birds-and-bees lecture, but most adolescents don't get to enroll in Masturbation 101. Instead, they turn to movies and pornographic films, which often feature a woman masturbating in stylized positions—usually on her back, so that her actions are visible to the camera, wearing high heels and in full hair and makeup. Typically, a man soon joins her. This rigid perspective on masturbation is discouraging, not least because it suggests that masturbation is only valid in conjunction with "real" sex.

It doesn't have to be. Masturbation is, literally, all about *your* pleasure. Before you give yourself a hand, so to speak, consider the ambience. Think of masturbation like a self-seduction: it might be a quickie, accomplished in minutes with your clothes on, or it could be an all-out showstopper.

Here are a few tips for getting in the mood.

Set the lighting so that it's flattering, relaxing, and comfortable. Light candles for a sensual, flickering glow.

Turn on music that you find sexy and arousing, whether it's rap, Beethoven's *Ninth*, or some dirty rock and roll.

Dress up for yourself. Why should you dress up only for your partner and let that cute lingerie collect dust in between romps? Throw on what *you* feel sexy in and admire yourself in the mirror before showing yourself some love.

SEXUAL COMMUNICATION

Communication isn't always easy. Here are some tips that'll make setting the sexual boundaries in your relationship a little smoother:

1. Make a "Yes, No, Maybe" list. Separately, you and your partner should each make a Y N M list. Write down which sex acts are totally okay with you; which acts are absolutely never going to happen, as far as you're concerned; and which ones you're willing to compromise on. Try this as an icebreaker—it's a great way to start the discussion. (Plus, you might be surprised at what both of you find negotiable.)

2. Be specific. Tell him exactly what you want when it comes to sex, and don't assume that he can read your mind or that he'll pick up on subtle hints. If you tell him that you want him to pay more attention to your breasts, be sure to tell him what you want him to do with your breasts—such as caress them while lovemaking, or complimenting you on them when you're wearing sexy lingerie or dressed up to go out.

3. Clarify your partner's responses so that he knows you're listening to him. This shows him, loud and clear, that you understand what he is saying. For example, "So, I understand that what you're telling me is, you expect us to make love at least once a week?"

4. Make the most of pillow talk. You and your partner are cuddled up and feeling cozy—before or after sex, maybe. Now is the time to ask him about his sexual personality, such as how often he masturbates, whether he enjoys porn, or how he fantasizes about sex. He might be more likely to be honest about his needs when he's feeling intimate—and you might, too. Plus, if you're feeling anxious about asking straightforward questions, doing so gently and sexily during pillow talk can help ease you into a more direct conversation.

5. Stay positive and avoid criticism. Just like basic communication skills, sexual communication skills thrive when you stay positive and focus on articulating your own thoughts and feelings, rather than blaming your partner for what he is or isn't doing. Use "I" statements instead of "you" statements. For instance, instead of saying, "You don't make me orgasm enough," try saying, "I feel excited when I know that you're trying to bring me to orgasm. I would love it if we could work on helping me finish."

6. Communicate what you like to him both verbally and physically. Tell him what you like about his lovemaking, and then tell him what else you'd like him to do. To really drive your point home, try *showing* him what you want. For example, maybe he already uses his mouth effectively on your clitoris, but you're dying for more G-spot stimulation. Say, "I love how you lick my clitoris. Let me show you another way you can touch me that drives me crazy." Then guide his hand between your legs and give him a personal introduction to your G-spot.

6. Compromise is king. While you should never compromise on things that are strictly no-go for you, you may want to consider compromising on acts that are important to your partner. If you want him to try new things that you like, it may help to show him that you're willing to give a little, too.

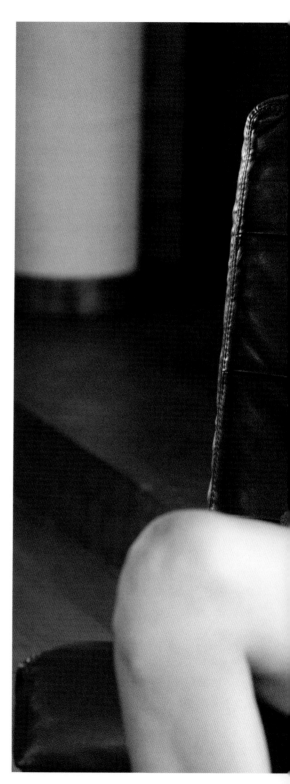

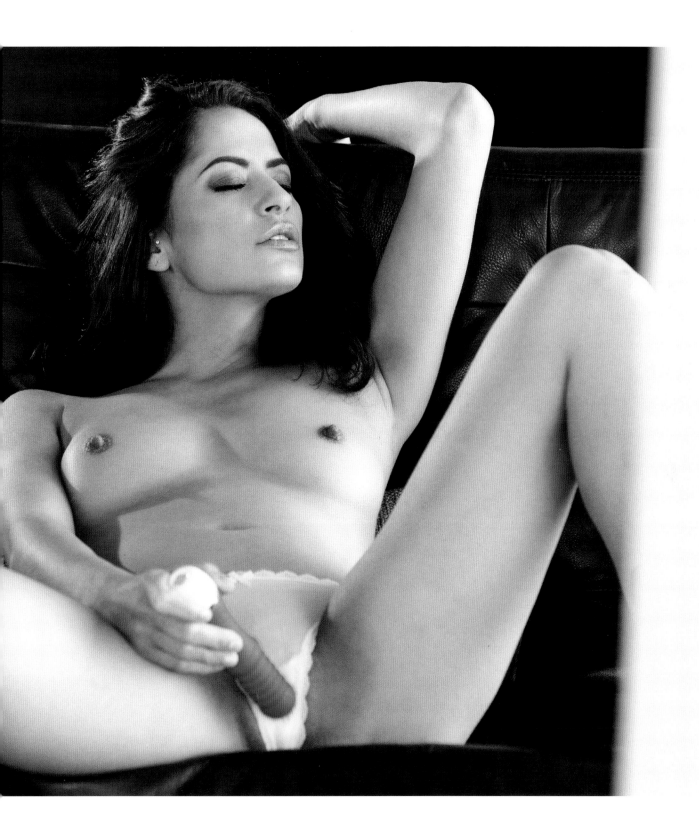

There's just one more thing to do before you get going: start thinking hot thoughts. Erotic thoughts and fantasies can act as your sexual guides as you start to touch yourself. Everyone's turned on by different things; go with whatever thoughts come to mind, and don't shame yourself for what comes naturally. Relax—this is a fantasy that you control. Summon thoughts of the exciting sexual experiences that you've had, and play the scenes out in your mind. Or let your thoughts wander into sexual situations you find attractive. Don't worry if ideas come to mind that you consider taboo. It's normal to be attracted to things that seem a little "wrong." Recently, at a conference, I sat in on a panel discussion with experts on women's sexuality. The panel included professors, physicians, psychologists, and even sex workers. During the question-and-answer session, an audience member asked the panel members to discuss their personal fantasies. Honestly and respectfully, each expert named her or his biggest secret fantasy. The lesbian academic researcher named an interracial heterosexual orgy, while the adult film star desired a romantic interlude with her husband. So let yourself go. This fantasy is just for you.

ASSUME THE POSITION

Now it's time to experiment. Don't feel limited to one position, technique, or style of self-love. There are an infinite number of ways to get yourself off, and there are no limits or rules. If you're new to it, though, you might try these positions:

1. Lying on your back. This creates a relaxing, easy way to access your vagina by using either your hands or sex toys.

2. Sitting up, or propped up, with a pillow. It's just as relaxing, but this position also allows you to look down at yourself, or to face a mirror so that you can watch the action.

3. Lying on your stomach. Lie facedown on your bed, the couch, or the floor. From here, it's easy to use your hands or a pillow to stimulate your clitoris or pubic mound by rubbing with a gentle pressure.

4. In the bath or shower. Lots of women love the sensation of warm water on the skin; it can provide additional stimulation to your clitoris and vulva. Many women swear by the pressure from an adjustable showerhead when it's aimed at the right places. Just be sure you don't spray water directly into the vagina as that can possibly cause an air embolism, which is rare but can be fatal. Simply use the shower to run water *over* your vagina and clitoris.

HANDY TECHNIQUES

Masturbation is all about enjoying the sensation of your own touch. Not sure how to start? Try these techniques—and then come up with a few of your own.

Rub your mound. Lie on your stomach with your hands between your bed and your pubic mound (that's the soft mound above your clitoris). Using gentle but firm pressure, rub your mound and experiment by rubbing in different directions, such as up and down, side to side, and in a circular motion.

Stimulate your clitoris. Start by using your index finger and your ring finger to part your labia. Use your middle finger to play with your clitoris. Trace circles on or around it, move your finger side to side or up and down—or do all of the above. (Or, if you're a first-timer and you find that your clitoris is too sensitive to touch directly, try placing a towel between your legs and then apply a little pressure.)

Start fingering. Use your index finger at first, then feel free to use any of your fingers while you're experimenting. Trace your fingers around your vulva and the surrounding area, moving them inward and in a circle when you feel ready to explore your vaginal opening. Slide your entire hand down your vulva and slowly slip your finger into your vagina. Notice its texture, moisture, and heat. Starting slowly, slide your finger in and out of your vagina at the pace that's most comfortable to you. Try other gestures, such as retracting your finger in a "come hither" motion while it's inside of you.

Use a toy. A dildo is a penis-shaped sex toy made to be inserted into your vagina, while a vibrator is a sex toy that vibrates—hence the name—in order to create clitoral stimulation. Many toys do both. Use a dildo—with lubrication, if necessary— while masturbating. It offers another level of penetration beyond your fingers. Most women enjoy using vibrators on and around the clitoris, and reach orgasm most easily this way. (For lots more on sex toys and how to choose one, check out chapter 10.)

Party with your G-spot. Using a toy or your fingers, find your G-spot. (Where's that again? Review my step-by-step instructions in chapter 1 if you're not sure.) Stimulate it through massage, pressure, and a variety of motions. For instance, insert your finger 1–2 inches (2.5–5 centimeters) into your vagina and press on the upper part of the vaginal cavity. Try a range of pressure levels, from light, regular pressure to forceful "pounding." Experiment to find out which motions and sensations really set your heart racing.

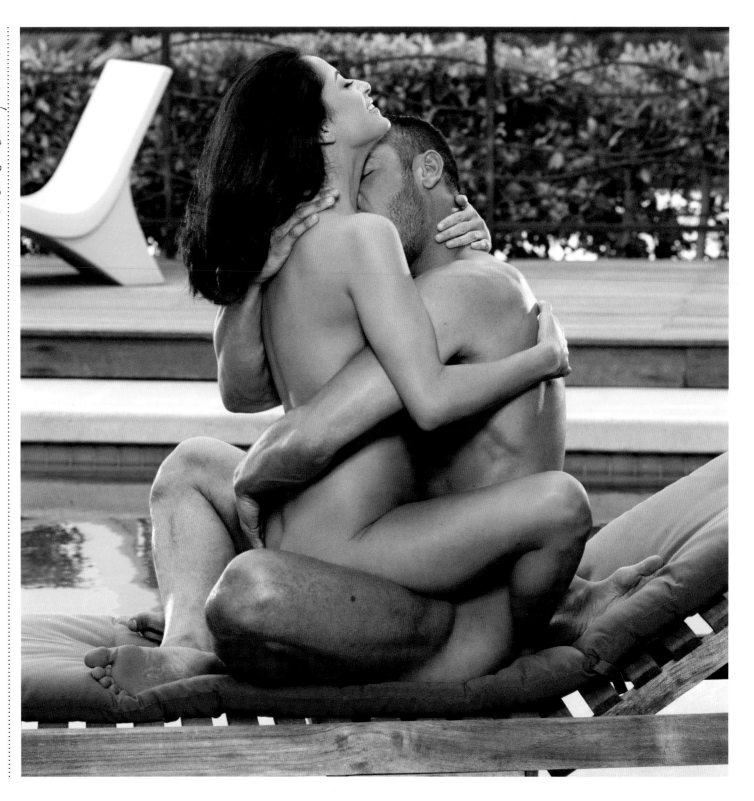

PLASTIC SURGERY: SHOULD YOU CONSIDER THE NIP AND TUCK?

Plastic surgery has become part of American culture. Prime-time reality TV shows can't get enough of it: some of them focus on celebrities who undergo the procedure, while others are based on women's so-called transformations through plastic surgery. Media like these place plastic surgery on a pedestal and convince viewers that surgery will identify them as elite, since it seems to go hand-in-hand with the famous, beautiful, and wealthy. Mommy makeovers, breast augmentation, and even labiaplasty encourage women to depreciate their most intimate sexual parts.

The fact is, as women, each one of us has the right to do what she likes with her body, and that includes a right to undergo elective plastic surgery. However—with the exception of medical issues that cause harm to yourself or others—there is certainly no *need* for you to surgically alter or augment your body. Before you go under the knife, take some time for self-examination. Why do you want surgery? Are you comfortable with its benefits and risks? Imagine that you're talking to your younger sister, daughter, or younger friend. What if she confided in you that she's planning on plastic surgery because she thinks her breasts are too small or too saggy, or that her labia are too long? What advice would you give her? If you'd advise her against it, ask yourself why you'd consider doing it yourself. If after careful reflection you're still thinking about plastic surgery, be sure to do the following:

1. *Educate yourself on the procedure.* Read books on it, view websites that detail it, and even watch videos of it in progress. Become familiar with the procedure, know its risks, and find out what to expect when you're healing.

2. *Research your plastic surgeon.* Ask for referrals from other patients, and look up your doctor's ratings. Don't go with the cheapest alternative: this is your body and your health, and now is not the time to cut corners.

3. *Consult your regular doctor.* Surgery is a major step even if done for cosmetic reasons. Be sure there aren't any underlying issues such as breast lumps, abnormal growths, heart or blood pressure inconsistencies, or allergies to medications that could make surgery risky.

4. *Work on yourself first.* If you're considering liposuction, set yourself a realistic period of time in which to focus on improving your figure through motivated healthy living. Then reevaluate.

5. *Try therapy.* With the guidance of a counselor or therapist, examine your reasons for being dissatisfied with your body. This is particularly recommended if you want multiple procedures. Are you sure that surgery will be a positive step toward self-acceptance?

If after educating yourself you still want to go forward, then do so. Own it. You are making a conscious decision with awareness of the risks and rewards. After all, it's your body, and it's your choice. It's important to know and love yourself—but if you've got those priorities in place, you should feel free to do what you please with your body.

COMMUNICATION AND BOUNDARIES: PROTECTING YOUR SEXUAL SELF-ESTEEM

Whether you're in a long-term relationship or enjoying casual sex on occasion, it's not always easy to talk about sex—even with your partner. Maybe you feel embarrassed or intimidated when you talk about it. If so, you're not the only one. Talking about sex raises lots of thorny issues, including STI test results, sexual values and expectations, and how often to have sex.

Setting sexual and emotional boundaries with your partner will help establish what you're comfortable with in the parameters of your specific situation. Never assume that your partner knows something that you haven't openly discussed. Talk about which sexual acts are okay with you, and which areas are no-go.

Make a "Yes, No, Maybe" list (see the sidebar on page 62) and use it as a tool to gauge where your boundaries are as a couple. It's really important to hear your partner talk about what sex means to him, and to communicate what it means to you. Perhaps you've started sleeping with a new partner: you may not be sleeping with anyone else, but that doesn't mean he's not. You won't know until you ask. Verbalize what sex means to you in terms of exclusivity. If you want to be sexually exclusive with your partner, you need to say it. You also want to know your partner's STI status, particularly if you're striking up a new sexual relationship, or if there's been a break in your monogamous relationship. Either way, being privy to your partner's test results is something you owe to yourself. I won't lie. "Do you have an STI?" is not an easy question to ask. But being polite won't seem important when you are looking at an STI diagnosis—and a compromised ability to have children and the burden of having to disclose that you have/had an STI to all future partners. Work toward feeling

more comfortable with bringing up the subject. Having this discussion ultimately protects your health and reproductive future.

Sexual self-esteem means loving yourself, first and foremost. And it's the most important way to make sex great for both of you. When you articulate your sexual needs and understand your own values and beliefs regarding sex, you'll be able to set boundaries and discuss sexpectations—even with casual partners. Better sex happens when you know and respect your unique sexual self. It's also intimately tied to the most important sex organ in your entire body: your brain. Keep reading to find out how your brain makes you the sexual being you are.

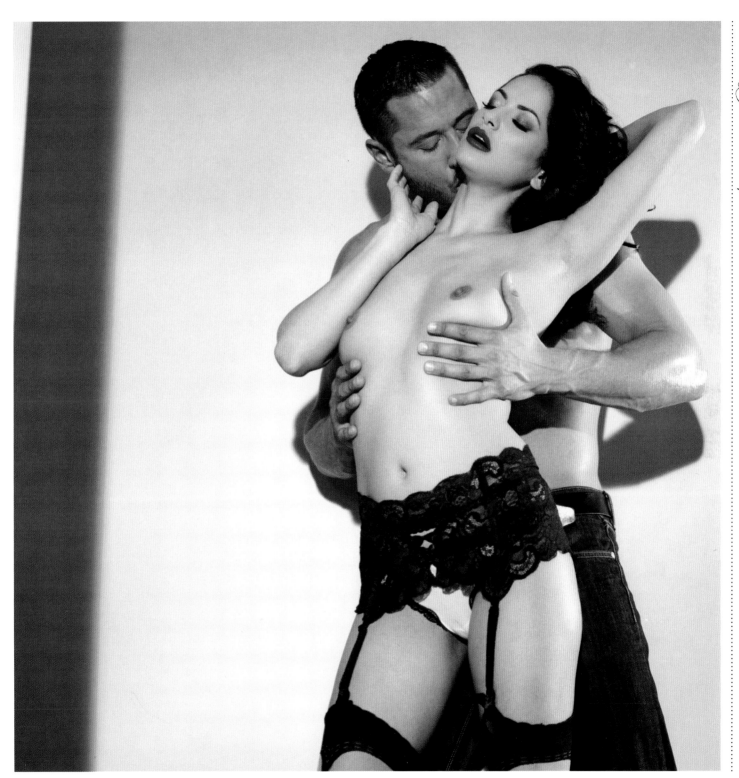

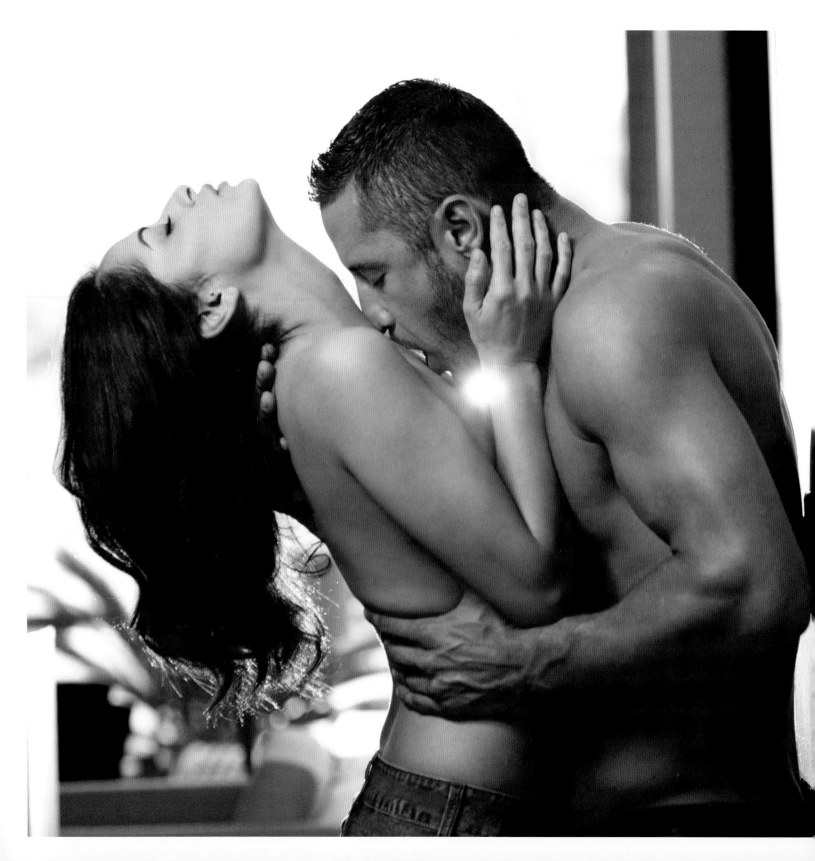

04 The Brain: Your Most Powerful Sex Organ

Although we might like to think that love and sex drive are mystical forces of nature, the fact is, we have our brains to thank. Chemicals called neurotransmitters, hormones, and other stimulants are responsible for a lot of our emotional and sexual responses. That said, we each have our own personal preferences when it comes to sex. This chapter is all about understanding your brain's relationship to your sex life. It'll help you understand and make the most of your own sexual responses, and will show you how to tune in to the differences between male and female sexual behavior. It'll explain the chemistry of attraction, and the impact your sex life has on your emotional and psychological well-being.

THIS IS YOUR BRAIN ON SEX

The brain is the most complex organ in the human body. Scientists are constantly finding new evidence of the brain's capabilities. For instance, neurologist Dr. Richard Davidson's research suggests that we can actually change both the function and the structure of our brains by undergoing certain experiences and emotions. The ability to change your brain function is called neuroplasticity, and it means that positive, healthy emotions aren't something you're born with—they can be learned. What's more, some studies have shown that learning or experience can also change the physical structure of the brain. One study, conducted at Harvard in 2000, investigated the ways in which short- and long-term meditation was able to alter the brain's activity levels in the areas that indicate anxiety, depression, anger, and fear, as well as the body's ability to heal itself. The results suggested that these changes in activity levels were due to structural plasticity—that is, to physical changes in the brain.

Of course, the brain has a powerful influence over an individual's actions, feelings, and thoughts. When it comes to sex and love, according to researcher Dr. Helen Fisher, the brain can be divided into three categories: sex, romance, and attachment. Each category is governed by a different network within the brain, with corresponding hormones and neurotransmitters.

Appetite for sex is controlled by the hypothalamus, the area of the brain that drives impulses like hunger and thirst. The hypothalamus also regulates the autonomic nervous system, which regulates unconscious body functions, such as heart rate and respiration. Meanwhile, if you're in the mood for romance, it's because neurotransmitters in your brain have been presented with a stimulus—that is, with a potential partner. (Neurotransmitters are chemicals that transmit signals within the brain.) MRI imaging studies have shown that the brains of the newly in love demonstrate a high amount of activity in the ventral tegmental area, which is located in the center of the brain. It becomes saturated with the neurotransmitters dopamine, cortisol, and norepinephrine, resulting in sensations of calmness and arousal, as well as the creation of short-term emotional memories.

That's why we experience that "high" feeling that always seems to accompany the first flush of romance. As for the desire for and drive toward attachment, it's fueled by the hormones oxytocin and vasopressin, both of which are secreted by the hypothalamus. These hormones give you a sense of well-being and make you want to bond with your partner.

Our experiences of lust, romance, and attachment—the three categories of love—often occur consecutively, as do the biological components that drive them. But that's not always the case. The order in which we experience them can change, and these categories can operate independently of one another, depending upon each person's individual mental and physical circumstances. What's more, while thoughts and emotions—or the release of

neurotransmitters—can cause behaviors to occur, the opposite is also true: changing your behavior can lead to a change in your thoughts and emotions. Therefore, spicing up the romance in your relationship can lead to greater attachment. (Neuroplasticity strikes again!) For example, you might not feel like having sex at first—but a little foreplay can put you in the mood pronto.

NEUROTRANSMITTERS AND HORMONES: THE KEYS TO EMOTIONAL AND SEXUAL SATISFACTION

Neurotransmitters and hormones become active during our experiences of sex and love, but they can also be released by other activities and behaviors. For example, exercise releases endorphins, dopamine, and serotonin into the bloodstream, making you feel calm and relaxed—just like that postsex glow. And serotonin is also a natural appetite suppressant, which means that doing regular exercise could make you less likely to overeat. That helps create a positive cycle of healthy living, which is vital to having great sex. Here are the neurotransmitters and hormones that help shape your sex life.

Dopamine

Dopamine is what stimulates you to work toward perceived rewards, like a promotion at work, a hug from (or great sex with!) your partner at the end of the day, or the ice-cream sundae you're treating yourself to at the end of a long week. Dopamine also makes you feel "high." That walking-on-clouds feeling you get after a great first date? Thank dopamine. It's responsible for that elated sense of well-being that keeps you flying postdate. (Addictive, dangerous drugs like methamphetamines and cocaine increase dopamine levels, too. Stay far, far away from them, and stick to the dopamine that your brain produces naturally.) Proper levels of dopamine in the brain ensure that your attention levels, focus, and short-term memory are sharp and clear.

Serotonin

A neurotransmitter that's found mostly in your stomach, serotonin helps regulate your mood, your appetite, and your sleep patterns. It also tends to be low in early romantic love. That's why, after a couple of great dates, you're thinking about him nonstop. You're ridiculously nervous. Will he text or call you? You obsessively check your phone, your email, and all your social media accounts every three minutes. Low serotonin levels are associated with anxiety, panic, and depression—and it's likely that early in a relationship, you'll show all the classic signs. The serotonin levels in your brain will rise as your relationship progresses and becomes long-term and committed. And that means you feel stable, serene, and convinced that your partner is the greatest guy in the world. Serotonin makes you want to get attached, and stay that way. Serotonin also contributes to feelings of well-being and happiness in general. When your serotonin levels are high, your mood lifts. You feel relaxed and tranquil, and you're likely to get a better night's sleep.

Oxytocin

A hormone that's produced by the pituitary gland, oxytocin is the cuddle chemical. Oxytocin stimulates feelings of attachment, and it's what causes mothers to bond with their newborn babies. It also encourages you to bond with your partner. It makes you feel calm around him, and it encourages you to trust him. And the more time

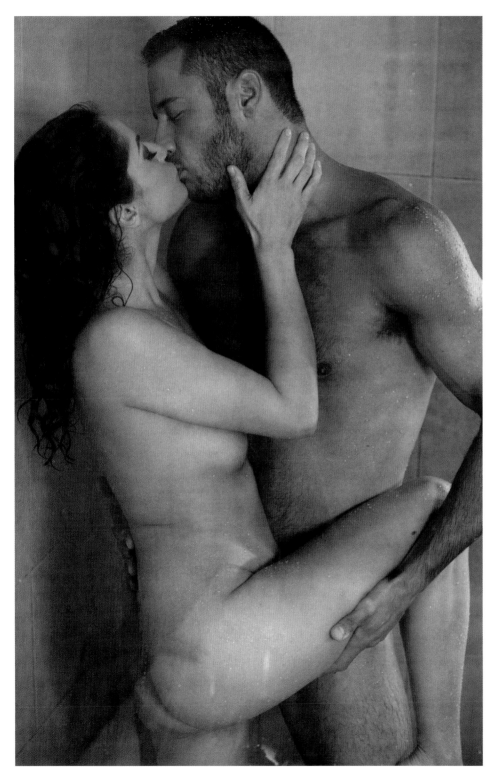

you spend with your partner, the more oxytocin your brain releases. Orgasm delivers a whopping dose of oxytocin to your brain. That's why you probably enjoy snuggling up with your partner for a while after sex. Like serotonin, oxytocin is associated with improved mood, decreased anxiety, and a sense of overall well-being.

Vasopressin
Like oxytocin, vasopressin is secreted by the pituitary gland, and it increases your desire to bond with your partner, since it increases after sex. Vasopressin makes you feel relaxed and tranquil after sex. It also helps you feel attached to your partner. It makes you more inclined toward monogamy and stokes your desire to stay with one mate instead of playing the field. The flip side of vasopressin is that it instills protectiveness—which can translate to jealousy. Vasopressin encourages both partners to protect each other and their offspring. It can also increase pain tolerance.

Adrenaline

Also known as epinephrine, adrenaline is responsible for the fight-or-flight reaction to stressful situations. But when it comes to sex, adrenaline also gets you excited. Adrenaline causes feelings of exhilaration, and causes your heart rate and blood pressure to increase before sex, preparing your body for the action.

Testosterone

It's common to think of testosterone as a male hormone, but the fact is, the sex organs of both genders produce it naturally. And it's a good thing, too, because testosterone is responsible for sexual arousal in both men and women. (But don't worry, you're not going to start sprouting a beard: women have about one-tenth to one-twentieth as much testosterone as men.) It makes your sex drive more intense and sexual behavior more assertive in both men and women.

Estrogen

It's the primary female sex hormone, but estrogen is present in both men's and women's bodies. In both genders, estrogen promotes bone strength and helps the body process cholesterol. It also helps you have better sex. While it doesn't actually increase your sex drive, estrogen has to be present for testosterone to work its libidinous magic. And its presence improves your vagina's elasticity and natural lubrication, making sex that much more pleasurable. Estrogen can also have a positive effect on mood and mental health. A decrease in estrogen levels—which can be brought on by menopause, or can occur postchildbirth—has been associated with depression, mood swings, and fatigue.

SNOOZING AFTER SEX

Now that you've gotten the rundown on the neurotransmitters and hormones that affect your sex life, what about that age-old question: why do men feel sleepy after sex?

1. Prolactin. When a man ejaculates, his body releases a protein called prolactin, which causes sexual satisfaction and a sense of calm. Thanks to high prolactin levels—which are four times higher after intercourse than masturbation—men can't become erect again right after sex. That temporarily dampens the libido.

2. Oxytocin, vasopressin, and serotonin. Produced after intercourse, the hormones oxytocin and vasopressin and the neurotransmitter serotonin promote bonding, affection, trust, and social relaxation, and also encourage that postsex sense of contentment.

3. Nitric oxide. After sex, nitric oxide is released through the prostate gland into the male body, and it affects the penis through the dilation of the blood vessels and muscle relaxation. This causes his erection to subside, and it reduces physical sexual tension.

4. Parasympathetic relaxation. You've enjoyed a great roll in the hay: now's when your parasympathetic nervous system kicks in to calm things down, create physical relaxation, and allow blood flow to return to the extremities. The fight-or-flight mentality is not present immediately after sex.

5. Physical exertion. If your partner is the one who's doing more of the physical "work" of sex, it's likely that he'll be more tired, sweaty, and drained than you'll be. Simply put, the physical demands of sex wear you out—in a good way.

KNOW THE THREE TYPES OF LOVE

Now you're down with brain chemistry's effect on that crazy little thing called love. But which roles do those chemicals play in our actual, day-to-day experiences of love? When it comes to the ways in which we experience emotion, it turns out that these chemicals help create very recognizable patterns. In fact, according to psychologist Robert Sternberg's triangular theory of love, intimate relationships usually fit one of three types: passion, intimacy, and commitment. Understanding these three emotions will help give you insight into your sexual relationship, whether it's a one-night stand, a budding relationship, or a committed marriage. Here's a rundown of the three types:

1. Lust, passionate love, or sexual attraction is a hormone-fueled craving for sexual gratification. When you first meet someone you like, you may feel an overwhelmingly intense sexual attraction to him. You might want to make love often, intimately, and anywhere or everywhere—especially in the beginning of the relationship. This kind of passion typically lasts a year or less. During this time, the body also releases the neurotransmitter phenylethylamine.

2. Intimacy, romantic love, or compassionate love is characterized by increased energy and focused attention, stimulated by dopamine, serotonin, and norepinephrine. Based upon mutual affection and understanding, this is the "bonding" kind of love that tends to hold relationships together.

3. Attached or committed love stimulates a sense of security, comfort, and emotional union, which is often demonstrated by actions like sharing meals, living together, sharing chores, and other affiliative behaviors. It also includes a mutual choice to be committed to one another. This type of love can exist apart from romantic love or passionate love, and is embodied by the elderly couple you might see enjoying one another's company on a park bench.

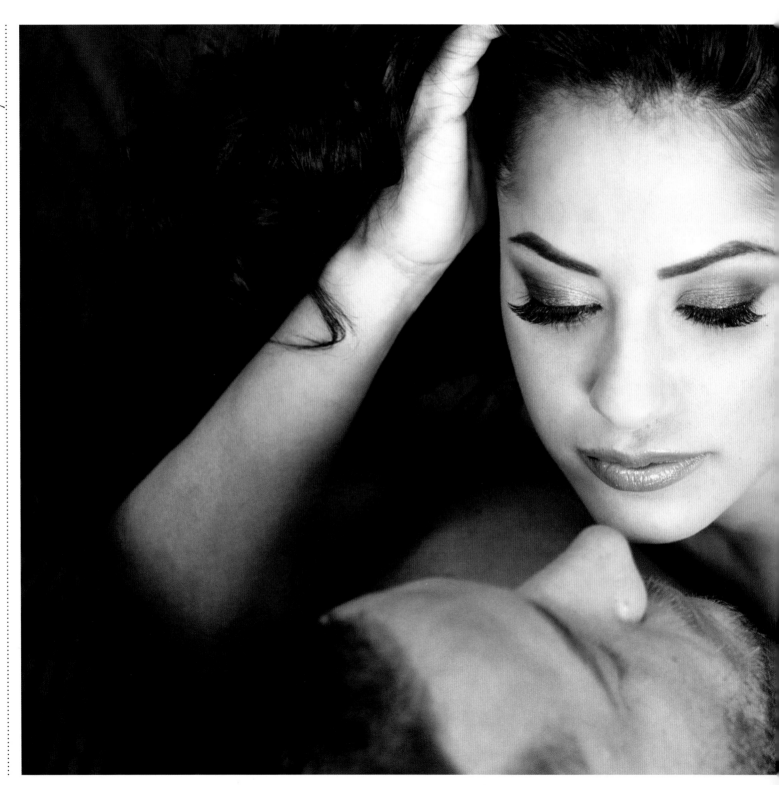

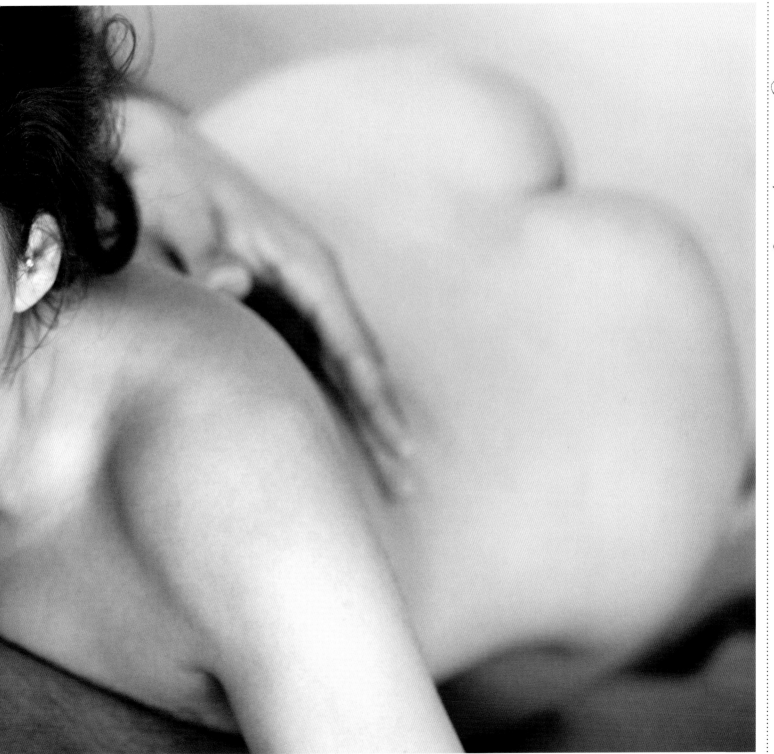

These three types of love can occur in combinations with each other, or completely separately. For example—as you probably know from experience—it's absolutely normal to fall head-over-heels in love with someone, to make love often, and to feel a strong attachment to him—only to have the relationship end platonically. After all, it takes effort and motivation to sustain passion, or restore the lust or spark back into an existing relationship. So, while lust is certainly exciting, the way you experience it may depend less on your new partner and more on your own brain chemicals. Or, you might feel lust for, and have sex with, a partner to whom you're not really attached. (And who hasn't?) You might even find yourself in "romantic" love with a partner with whom you're not in a sexual relationship. The moral of the story is, there are many different types of interactions within the scope of love, and it's up to you to choose which is right for you, and when.

THE CHEMISTRY OF ATTRACTION

Attraction is, of course, the falling-in-love phase, or the experience of being infatuated with another person. Flooded by hormonal stimulants, including dopamine, norepinephrine, and phenylethylamine, the brain becomes awash with euphoria, which makes us feel like we've been swept away by our emotions. After a while, though, your body's tolerance for these chemicals increases, and, as time passes, it produces less of these stimulants. That leaves some people craving another "hit"—which explains why some people become "attraction junkies," seeming to move from partner to partner every few months. That elusive high feeling simply fades after the initial stimulation is over. (However, it's also true that the high can return if both partners make an effort. Some couples describe their relationship as falling in and out of love over time.)

Some studies have proved what the perfume industry has always known: the experience of attraction can also be triggered by scents. Pheromones, or chemicals released by the body that are perceived by scent, may cause behavioral changes in others and can play an important role in attraction. They're present in bodily fluids such as male sweat and female vaginal secretions, and might be partly responsible for our choice of sexual partners.

A psychological research model called imprinting takes these powerful physiological dimensions into account. It considers the ways we experience intimate relationships—and decide whom we find attractive—by examining the interactions between our genetic makeup, our hormonal shifts, and the psychological experiences of our lives. Together, these components guide us (unconsciously, of course) when we choose intimate partners. You might hear people say that opposites attract, but studies have shown that the opposite cliché is in fact true: birds of a feather flock together. Scientifically, you're more likely to be attracted to someone similar to yourself.

BATTLE OF THE SEXES: THE DIFFERENCES BETWEEN MEN'S AND WOMEN'S BRAINS

Men are from Mars, and women are from … well, you know. Dozens of books have been written about the ways in which the two sexes try to unravel each other's mysteries. Too often, men and women have unrealistic expectations when it comes to one another's behavior. The reality is that men and women think differently due to biological structural differences in the brain as well as cultural norms, and we need to accept that. Try to tune in to the way the male brain works, and do make an effort to communicate with your partner about what he is thinking and feeling.

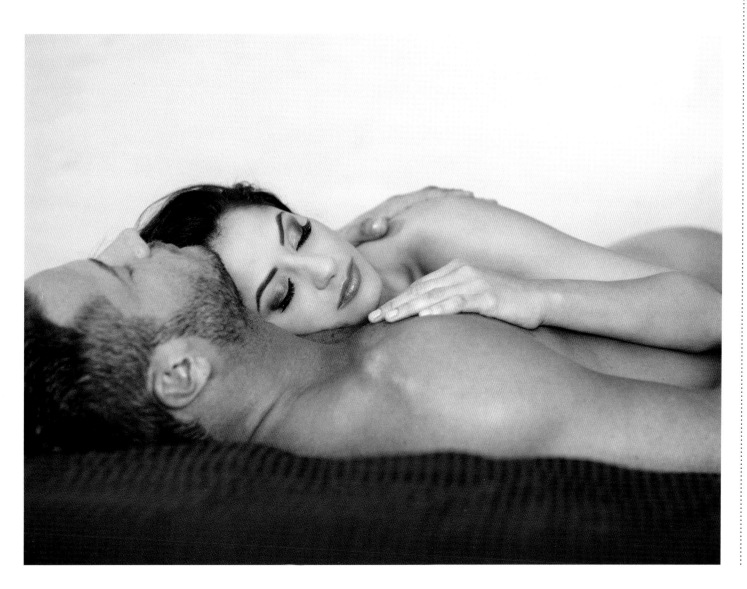

So, how are men and women different when it comes to sex? Let me blind you with science for a moment.

First, there are basic differences in the physical biology of the brain in areas related to sex. The preoptic hypothalamus is twice as big in men as it is in women. This is the area that controls the release of sex hormones in the pituitary glands. Another difference between the male and female brain is that men have a sexual pursuit area that is over two times larger than the one in the female brain.

Second, men respond to different sexual stimuli. Men are more responsive to visual stimulation than women. This might be why you'll notice men staring when an attractive woman (like you!) walks by. It's also why men get so turned on by lingerie, cleavage, and other easily visible sexual stimuli. Women, on the other hand, are more interested in experiences that involve connection and emotion. We have a broader spectrum of sexual stimuli, which is why women report bisexuality more often than men do. It's also why women generally have greater variations in sexual fantasies, and experiment more often with the opposite sex than men do.

Third, men define intimacy differently. Men tend to define intimacy by what they do with a partner when they're side by side with one another, like taking a walk or watching television. (This might be why men report feeling close to their partners when they watch television together, while women often don't regard it as quality time spent together.) Women, conversely, define intimacy by face-to-face engagements, such as having a conversation or sharing a meal. So, treat your partner to some male-friendly intimacy by having dinner sitting side by side rather than across from each other.

Fourth, men and women are hormonally different. For example, each gender responds differently to the hormone oxytocin. A recent study has shown that while oxytocin helped women better identify familial relationships, it helped men identify competitive relationships. This means that a man may feel and act protectively toward his partner as he becomes attached to her, while a woman might be likely to focus on family connections and togetherness as her relationship with her partner grows.

THE CHOICE IS YOURS

All this isn't to say that we're slaves to biology, or that our sex lives are at the mercy of hormones and neurotransmitters. Culture plays a big role, too. Since the rules of attraction, sexuality, and appropriate romantic behavior vary among cultures, you probably have built-in, culturally designated criteria when it comes to choosing a sexual partner, on top of your physiological drives. So while your choices are, to some extent, influenced by biological and cultural factors, it's still your prerogative—and your responsibility—to actively and consciously choose the partner that's right for you. For instance, you might feel a surge of lust when you meet a hot guy at a bar, but that doesn't mean you have to sleep with him—unless you want to. It's okay to weigh your sexual options, and to choose the one that's right for you, right now.

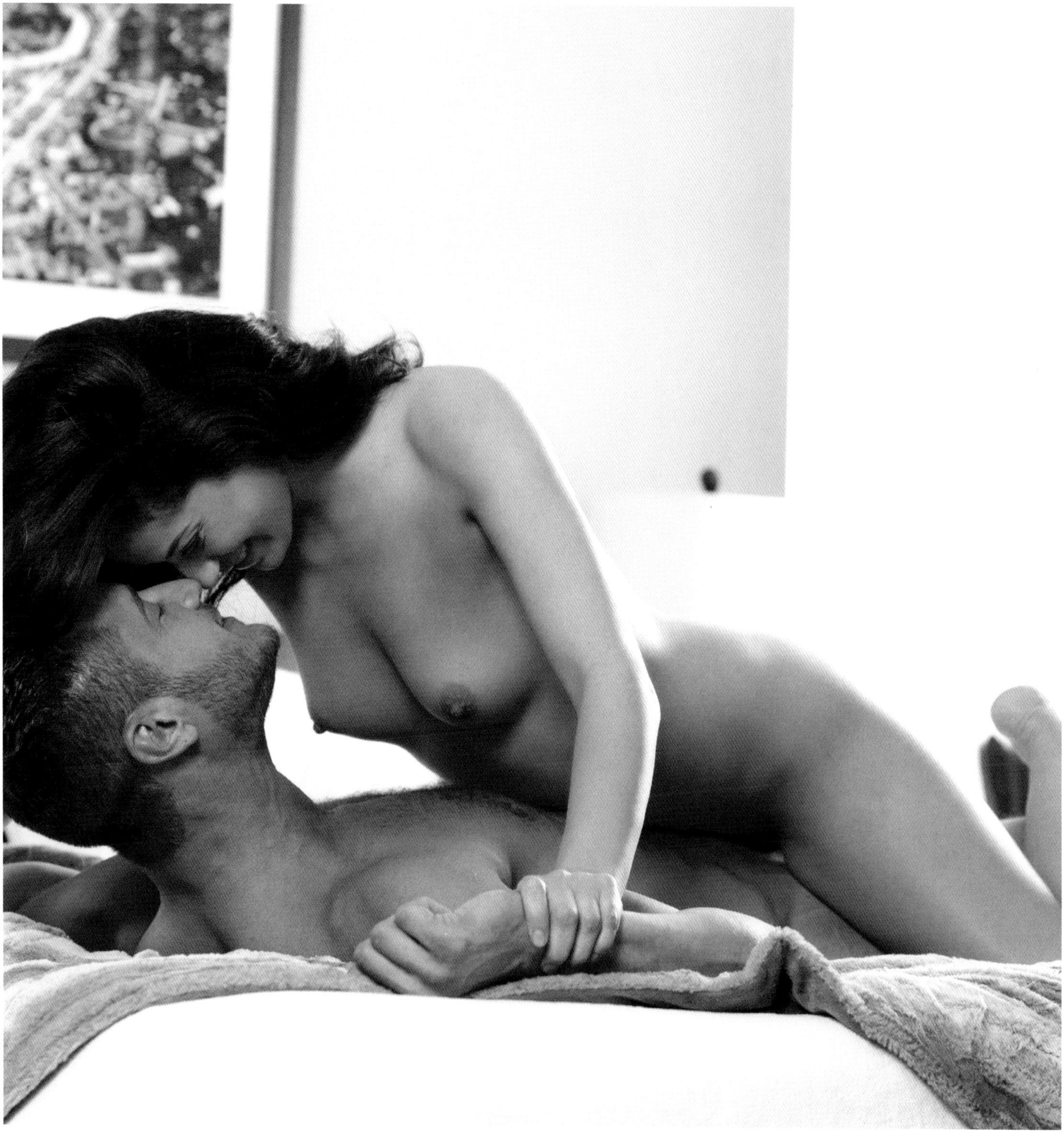

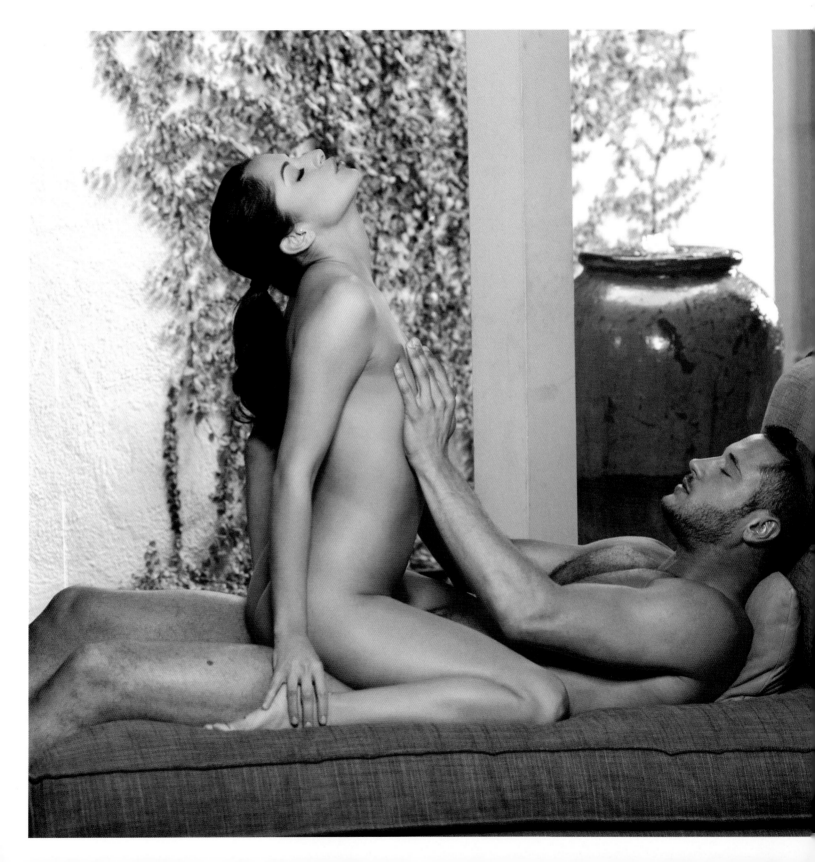

05 | *Orgasms: Getting to the Big "O"*

Lots of us think of sex as a race. How soon can he get it up? How soon can we get it on? How quickly can I come? Thanks to the movies and other media, we expect "good" sex to happen fast and to end in orgasm—every time. (Flash to the scene of the happy couple lying in bed with a snow-white sheet pulled up to their chins, saying, "That was great!") Reality looks a bit different. If you think of orgasm as sex's magical finish line, it might be time to change your perspective on sex and orgasms. Let's debunk a few orgasm-related myths first.

IT'S A MARATHON, NOT A SPRINT

Whether you're a competent comer or a first-timer when it comes to orgasms, this chapter will give you the lowdown on how orgasms work (and why faking it doesn't). It'll show you how to have multiple orgasms (all women can do it!), and will spill the beans on the sex positions that are most likely to help you reach the big O. Let's take a look at some orgasm myths.

I can't have an orgasm. Orgasms are possible for all women (with the exception of some rare biological instances—and it's unlikely you're one of them). Each woman experiences orgasm at a different age, speed, and with a different style of penetration or stimulation. If you've never had an orgasm, or if your orgasms are infrequent, know that it's not just you: about one-third of women report that they rarely have orgasms.

My partner should be able to make me come. Cultural expectations imply that if a man works hard enough, he should be able to make his partner orgasm. And lots of those expectations center on his penis. But the fact is, the duration of your partner's erection, his style of penetration, and his penis size are irrelevant to how you reach orgasm. While men typically orgasm and ejaculate following stimulation of the penis by a rhythmic stroking motion, women's experiences are often very different. For women, sex and orgasms don't necessarily occur in this step-by-step fashion.

Women can only have clitoral orgasms. The truth is, women can orgasm from either clitoral or vaginal stimulation—or a blend of the two—and we can experience different types of orgasmic sensations as a result. The pleasure women enjoy during sex tends to build up in a gradual, satisfying crescendo, as opposed to a more intense spike during orgasm, as with men. Women may or may not ejaculate (yes, women *can* ejaculate), but whether or not you ejaculate has nothing to do with the sensation or intensity of your orgasm.

FAKING IT ISN'T WORTH IT

According to a study published in the *Journal of Sex Research* in 2010, 67% of heterosexual women admitted to having faked an orgasm on at least one occasion—while only 20% of men suspected that a woman had faked an orgasm while being in bed with them. That means that the majority of American women are doing a great job of pretending they've climaxed—and, simultaneously, have really pumped up their guys' egos. (With hot air, that is.) While faking an orgasm might relieve the psychological pressure to hurry up and get off, faking it may have some long-term negative repercussions for your ability to orgasm—and, ultimately, your ability to connect with your partner. From a psychological perspective, avoidance—in any life circumstance—causes you to be *more* fearful of the thing you're avoiding, not less. By faking an orgasm now, you're actually preventing yourself from being able to easily have a real orgasm with your future partners.

So why do we do it? The main reasons that women fake orgasms, in order of frequency, include:

1. *Pleasing their partners.* "I know he loves it when I come."

2. *Feeling pressure to hurry up and finish.* "He came first, but I'm just not there yet. It's going to take way too long. Let's just wind things up."

3. *Avoiding hurting their partners' feelings.* "If I don't orgasm, will he feel like he's to blame? I don't want him to think he did anything wrong."

4. *Being tired.* "I'm just too exhausted to be into it tonight—and I've got way too much on my mind. Time to get this over with."

5. *Being bored.* "What he's doing really isn't working for me, and I'm losing interest—fast. If he thinks I've come, maybe he'll stop beavering away down there."

What's alarming is that two of these reasons—including the most frequent of them—are centered around the man's sexual pleasure and his psychological gratification. Historically, women have been taught to be submissive rather than aggressive when it comes to sex: we've been encouraged to defer to the needs of male sexuality, instead of articulating our own. Happily, that's changed. Most men are genuinely pleased when they know that you're feeling pleasure during sex. So, instead of faking an orgasm, try talking to your partner about what turns you on and what he can do to help you come. (It's okay to be nervous: talking about your sexual needs with your partner can be a little scary—or cringe-inducing—the first time, but it'll get easier and easier with practice. I promise.) If you find yourself getting bored during sex, take matters into your own hands. Tell him that spending a long time down there working at it, so to speak, doesn't necessarily mean that you'll get off. Then show him where you want to be touched. Don't be afraid to masturbate in front of him. Your partner will love watching you make yourself climax: a woman who knows her body and can orgasm by herself is sexy and empowered.

THE FOUR-STAGE SEXUAL RESPONSE CYCLE: THE MECHANICS OF YOUR ORGASM

While there are differences in the ways men and women experience sexual pleasure, patterns in sexual response in both men and women show that there are some general similarities between the two genders when it comes to reaching orgasm. For both, sexual arousal and response are not simply limited to the genitals. In fact, the entire body and mind work together in creating and experiencing a climax.

According to William Masters and Virginia Johnson, pioneers in sexual research who began their studies in the late 1950s, sexual response in both men and women develops in four stages:

1. *Excitement phase.* During the excitement or arousal stage, blood flow to the pelvic area increases, causing erections in men and vaginal lubrication in women. That means your vaginal area physically changes. Your clitoris swells, your vagina becomes wet and lubricated, and your labia thicken. Your skin might become flushed. Your breasts might swell, and your nipples may become erect. Your muscles tense, your heart rate increases, and your blood pressure rises.

2. *Plateau phase.* It's more exciting than it sounds! The plateau phase is the stable, leveled-off phase in which arousal is maintained. (By the way, a longer plateau phase often means more enjoyable sex.) The action has started, and you're into foreplay or having intercourse. You'll notice more changes in your vagina: your clitoris retracts under the clitoral hood, your vagina expands, and your labia become swollen and red. Your uterus elevates, your breasts continue to swell, and your breathing, heart rate, and blood pressure will increase even more as you get ready to come.

3. *Orgasm.* The rush of physical pleasure associated with the release of sexual tension can last anywhere from a few seconds to one minute. Once you reach climax, a number of different muscular contractions kick in. You'll feel rolling contractions in your uterus, and you might experience some loss of muscle control, such as minor muscle spasms. Respiration, heart rate, and blood pressure will be at their peak.

4. *Resolution phase.* After you orgasm, your body moves into the resolution phase. Now, your clitoris returns to its normal size, and your vagina relaxes. Your uterus returns to its normal position, while your cervix widens for about thirty minutes. Your labia and breasts become less flushed, your muscles relax, your heart rate decreases, and your breathing slows.

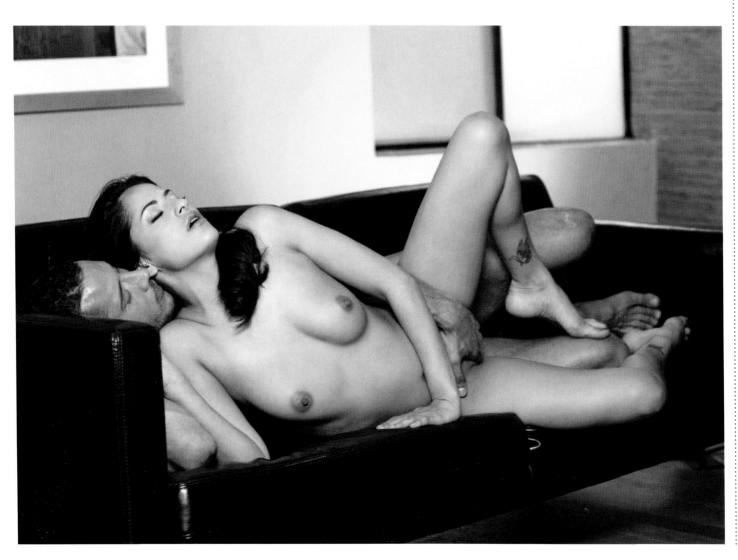

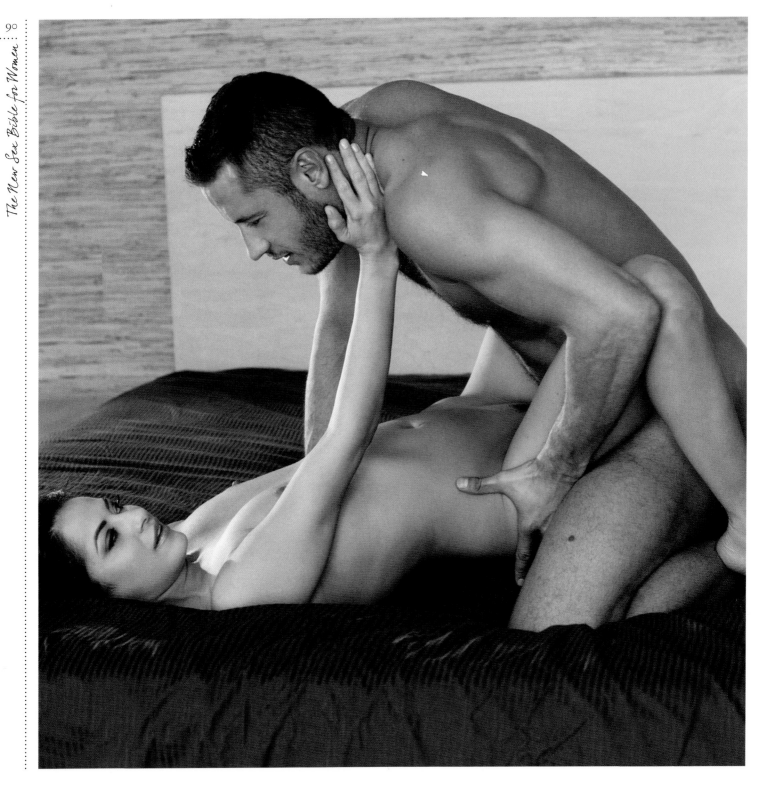

GETTING TO YES: THE THREE TYPES OF ORGASM

Sometimes being a woman has its perks. One of those perks is the fact that women can experience three different types of orgasms: clitoral, vaginal, and blended orgasms. (Aren't you glad you're not a man?)

Clitoral orgasms are the result of direct stimulation of the clitoris, which can be done manually, orally, or using a vibrator. For most women, clitoral orgasms are the easiest type of orgasm to achieve, whether alone or with a partner. (There are about eight thousand nerves in that tiny button-sized mound we call the clitoris.) The reason many women find it difficult to orgasm during penetrative sex is because there's typically no direct stimulation to the clitoris during vaginal sex. But there's a simple solution. Use your fingers or a toy, such as a vibrator, to give your clitoris a little attention during intercourse—or you can even show your partner how to stimulate it during sex. You can also try switching sex positions. Some moves, such as getting on top of him, do provide some clitoral stimulation.

Vaginal orgasms occur from G-spot stimulation, and some women find them harder to achieve. Why? You're less likely to come during vaginal intercourse or penetration due to the lack of nerves in the vaginal canal. Next time you have sex or masturbate with a toy you can insert into your vagina—such as a dildo—pay attention to the way penetration feels. While you may feel pleasure and pressure, you won't experience the heightened sensations you feel when you stimulate your clitoris. Still, don't let this fool you into thinking that the vagina isn't sensitive: it is. Some areas of the vulva, such as the labia, are very sensitive, and the pressure and friction of penetration can be really pleasurable. Then, of course, there's your G-spot. Located on the roof of your vagina, your G-spot might feel like a walnut, or the firm-but-spongy tip of your nose. Placing pressure on the G-spot can cause vaginal orgasms—and, in some cases, female ejaculation. Want to have more vaginal orgasms? Try using a toy that's angled upward to make stimulating your G-spot easier. Or experiment with your fingers and different sex positions. For instance, try getting on top or placing a pillow under your hips to lift them while you're in the missionary position. (Need a quick refresher course? There's lots more information on finding and loving your G-spot in chapter 1.)

A *blended orgasm* is a combination of vaginal and clitoral orgasms. It's less common than separate clitoral and vagina orgasms, but it's certainly possible (and *very* pleasurable). Different positions and techniques work for different women, but try this one: get on top of him, and circle his penis with your hips at the angle that stimulates your G-spot while rubbing your clitoris at the same time.

MULTIPLE ORGASMS

Essentially, a blended orgasm means having two orgasms at once. What about having two orgasms in a row? It's doable. Men have a postsex refractory period that prevents them from having multiple orgasms, but women don't. That means it's perfectly possible, biologically speaking, for women to have multiple orgasms. The trick, it seems, is to stay aroused and keep the stimulation going. Sexologists Masters and Johnson reported that women are capable of achieving additional orgasms if they are restimulated immediately following an orgasm, and if arousal levels have not dropped below the plateau phase. And it pays off: after the first orgasm, additional orgasms may feel more intense, and may be longer in duration. Once you can reach orgasm alone through masturbation and with a partner, you can do it, too.

To start becoming multiorgasmic, try these steps:

1. Extend your foreplay. By increasing the time it takes you to become fully aroused, you'll ensure that your body is ready to orgasm. Be mindful of the physical changes that occur when your body's aroused, such as lubrication levels. Move into penetrative sex only when you feel you're as turned on as possible.

2. Don't hit it and quit it. Many women feel so sensitive and exhausted after their first orgasm that they pull away from their partner or revert to cuddle mode. If you're in the mood for multiples though, try not to take too much downtime: you're more likely to reach a second orgasm if you try again right after the first time you climax. So instead of getting out of bed or cuddling right away, take a minute (or even less) to recover and connect with each other and then move toward another orgasm. Try deep kissing, slow oral sex, licking, or caressing, and then try penetration again. That'll help you get your second wind.

3. Stay in the moment. Try not to let your mind wander. (That does happen naturally during sex—but now is the time to stay focused!) Be in the moment and pay attention to your aroused body. Think about how your skin feels, how swollen and sensitive your vulva feels, and what his body feels like next to yours. Staying in the moment psychologically will help you keep the arousal level up as you move toward round two.

4. Vary the technique and type. For instance, if your first orgasm was clitoral and came from manual or oral stimulation, attempt a vaginal or G-spot orgasm for the second round. The changes in sensation will keep you aroused and excited.

5. Stay motivated. Once you're able to achieve an orgasm, even if it's during masturbation, you *are* capable of reaching multiple orgasms. That's a fact. As with any sexual situation, just relax, and listen to your body.

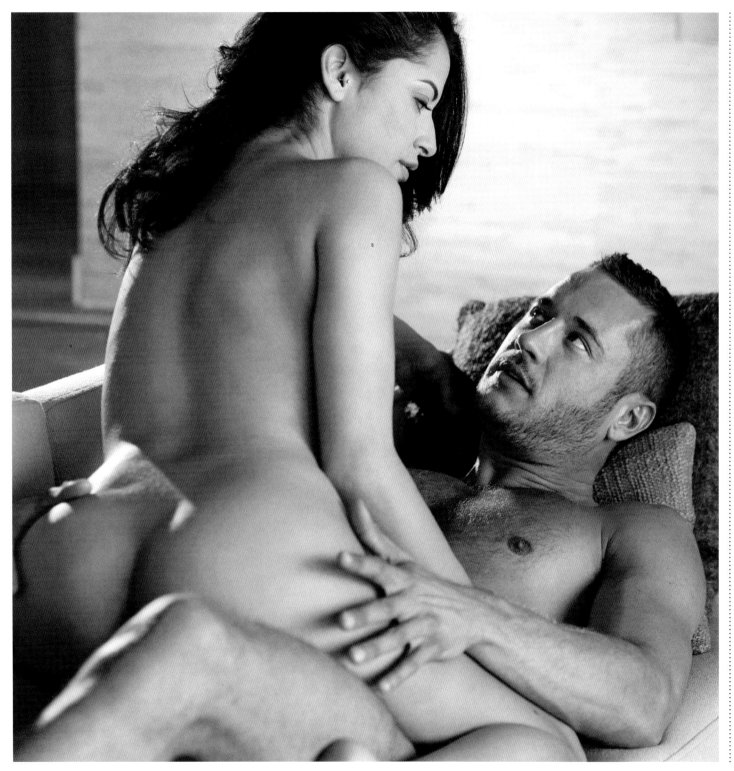

FEMALE EJACULATION: TRUE OR FALSE?

Female ejaculation has become a hot topic, and everyone from feminist scholars to the medical community has an opinion. So what's the real story? The fact is, all women have the biological structures necessary for ejaculation, but, due to individual differences such as anatomy, body knowledge, pelvic floor muscle strength, and ability to relax, not everyone has experienced it.

The origin of, reason for, and mechanics of the female ejaculation are still being studied and researched, so there's a lot to be learned about it. (In fact, until the 1980s, female ejaculate was regarded as a form of urine.) Today, the medical community agrees that female ejaculation exists, but the details are fuzzy. Here's what we know:

The fluid is released by the Skene's glands, which are located around the lower part of the urethra.

The amount of fluid released during female ejaculation can be as little as a teaspoon or as much as one cup.

Female ejaculate is not urine!

Women's bodies may have developed this function in order to prevent urinary tract infections.

Typically, it happens as a result of G-spot stimulation, in sexual positions such as woman-on-top or rear-entry.

Many women who experience ejaculation aren't expecting it and can't control it. It doesn't mean that the sex was exceptionally good, and it doesn't have anything to do with how powerful or meaningful her orgasm was. In one study, about 60% of women said that they'd felt some type of fluid release, whether "ejaculate" or not, during orgasm; 13% of women reported that they had experienced ejaculation at some point; and only 6% reported that it happens to them frequently. So, most women will have some experience with female ejaculation, to one degree or another.

Some women who've experienced female ejaculation say they feel ashamed or embarrassed, especially when it comes to their partners' reactions. Does this sound familiar? If so, know that you have the right to be proud of your body: after all, ejaculation is simply how your body responds positively to a sexual experience. Tell your partner what's happening to your body, and that it's one of many signs that you were enjoying yourself with him. And don't get down on yourself if you've never ejaculated. If you'd like to increase the likelihood of ejaculating, there are a few things you can do, including staying relaxed during sex, building strong pelvic floor muscles through Kegel exercises, and—most important—directly stimulating your G-spot during sex, through woman-on-top and rear-entry positions.

HOW TO COME MORE OFTEN—AND MORE INTENSELY

Maybe you're struggling to reach orgasm—or maybe you've been climaxing easily for years. Either way, these tips will help you get there easily, and more often. Here's your orgasm toolbox:

Focus on the clitoris and the G-spot. When it comes to coming, this is prime real estate.

Relax, and understand that sometimes, climaxing takes time. Some women can orgasm in a minute, while others need twenty minutes of stimulation and foreplay. Get to know your body and set realistic expectations for yourself.

Masturbate, masturbate, masturbate. It's so important to get to know your body, and to find out what makes you climax. Do a little self-help before you work on getting there with a partner.

Know your turn-ons. Get to know what turns you on and keeps you in the mood. Each woman has her own "go-to" fantasies and sensations that keep her moving toward orgasm.

Mix it up. While on top, use the movement of your hips in different ways to stimulate your G-spot. For example, try grinding or circling rather than moving up and down.

Multitask. Try two forms of stimulation at once. Try rubbing your clitoris while you're on top. Or, while he's going down on you, have him stimulate your G-spot with his finger at the same time.

Check the calendar. You'll be more likely to orgasm during the middle of your menstrual cycle, when you're ovulating. That's because your body's estrogen levels increase during this time, which, typically, also means an increase in sex drive. You're also more likely to get pregnant during this time, so make sure your birth control or protection is at hand—then get it on.

Pick your partners wisely. If you're not comfortable with your partner, it's likely that you won't be able to relax and focus on your own body.

Keep trying—the trying is the fun part, after all! If you do get there, be proud of yourself. As sexual women, our bodies are a little less "mechanical" than men's, so we may need a little more time, stimulation, and focus to come. When you do get there, notice what brought you to orgasm—and, of course, enjoy the moment.

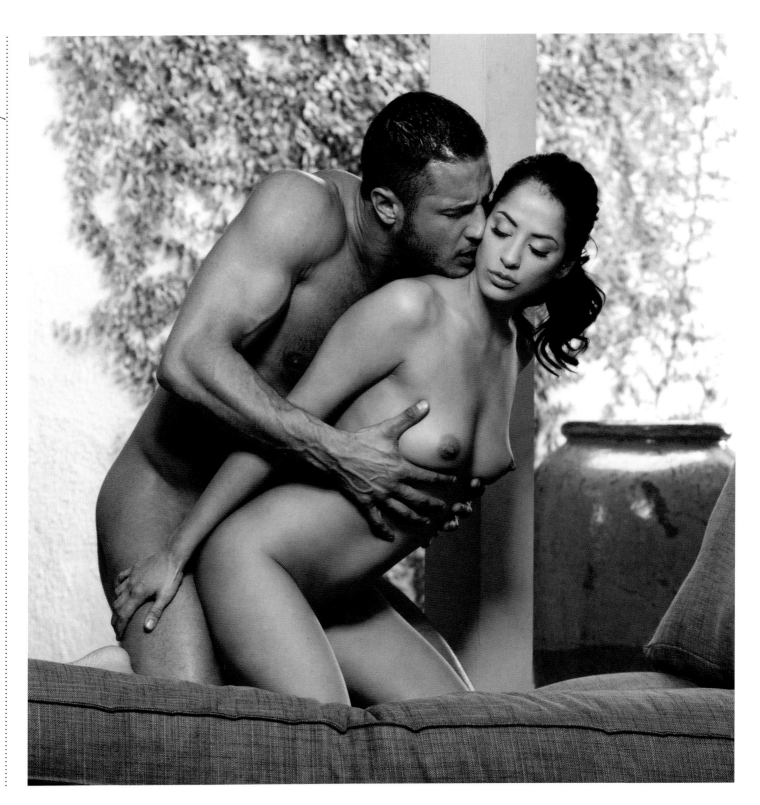

PROBLEMS REACHING ORGASM?

About 10% of women have never had an orgasm, and many women find climaxing difficult due to medical, biological, or psychological factors. Of the women who aren't having orgasms, about 95% are considered to be preorgasmic—that is, capable of reaching orgasm. As always, if you're having ongoing trouble reaching orgasm, it's best to consult with your doctor (preferably a gynecologist whom you like and trust).

Difficulty climaxing can be caused by medical issues, such as side effects from medications, health conditions related to nerves or hormones, or illnesses that impact your physical ability to be sexual. That's why it's important to talk to your doctor. You might be able to switch medications or modify dosages in order to reduce sexual side effects.

Biological issues can also make climaxing difficult. For example, vaginismus is a disorder that causes a woman's vaginal muscles to tighten when an object approaches the vagina—kind of like how your eye automatically closes when something comes near it. This physical reaction can be caused by a variety of circumstances, from psychological trauma to hyperactive pelvic floor muscles. Dyspareunia, or painful intercourse, can also prevent orgasm, and it can be caused by physical or psychological concerns. If you think you might be suffering from conditions like these, make an appointment with your doctor to discuss treatments, which range from vaginal hormone creams to vaginal dilators.

Sometimes, orgasm is difficult for psychological reasons. If you're anxious about or dissatisfied with your relationship, you might not be able to focus on your own pleasure during intercourse. Or, if you're a victim of abuse or trauma, intimacy and sexuality might trigger subconscious responses to your trauma. It might be helpful to check in with a therapist, especially one who specializes in sexuality, to explore your concerns.

BEST SEX POSITIONS FOR THE BIG "O"

Ultimately, you can make any sex position work to your benefit and orgasm during it. (Check out chapter 7 for a guide to lots of them.) That said, here are three top orgasm-inducing sex positions for you to try tonight:

1. *Modified Missionary with Elevated Hips.* By elevating your hips during missionary position, you'll create the perfect angle for G-spot stimulation. For maximum pleasure, rub your clitoris with your finger at the same time.

2. *Woman on Top.* Being on top gives you the stimulation and control that you need—and it gives him a great view of your entire body in the throes of pleasure. While you're on top, stimulate your clitoris by leaning slightly forward and grinding on him in an oval motion, rather than just moving up and down on his penis. This oval motion will allow his penis—regardless of shape and size—to hit your G-spot.

3. *Rear Entry.* When he enters you from behind, you'll be able to stimulate your clitoris by hand while his penis is at the perfect angle for G-spot stimulation. Another variation is lying flat on your stomach and using your body pressure to grind onto your hand for additional clitoral pressure. Start on your hands and knees and have him enter you from behind. Then slowly straighten your knees, stretch out your arms, and flatten yourself on the bed. Have him continue penetration on top of you. (It'll be easiest for him if he holds himself straight up on his arms.)

Having great orgasms requires one major thing: practice. Enjoy it! Find out what turns you on, both solo and with a partner, and then do it again (and again and again). Soon, you'll be able to get yourself off just about anytime. As the saying goes, you won't make it if you fake it—so don't bother. Instead, focus on working toward orgasm and loving the process. Read on to find out how knowing the ins and outs of his body can make sex that much hotter for you both.

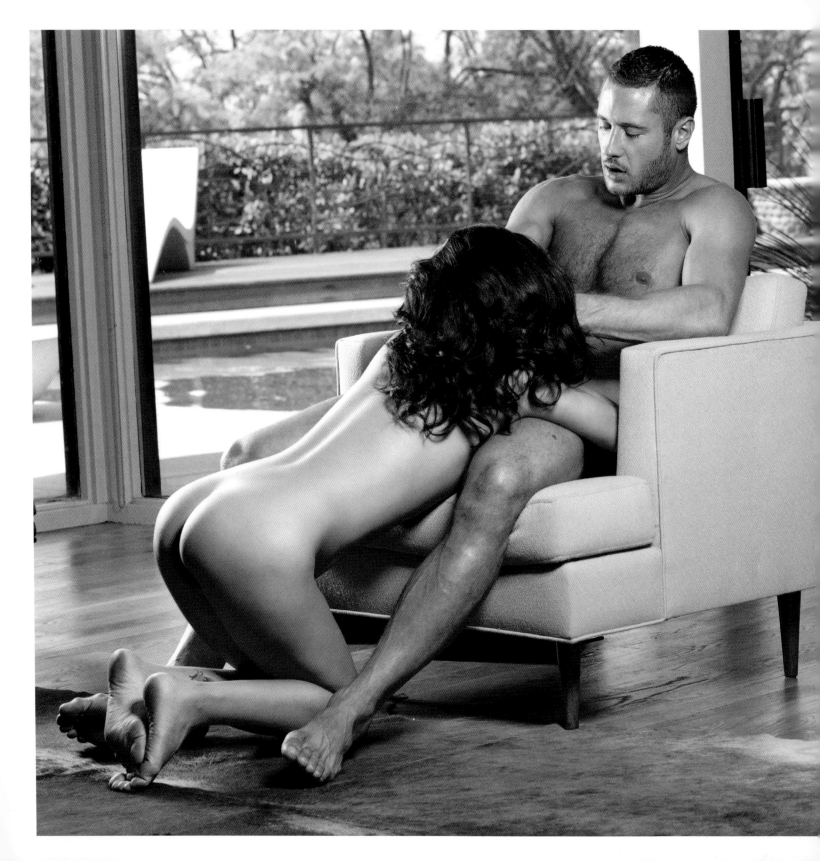

06 *The Male Body: His Pleasure, Your Pleasure*

The male body experiences sex and sexual pleasure differently than the female body, and as an intrepid sexual explorer, it's important that you know the territory into which you're venturing. Understanding the sexual ins and outs of the male body will help you feel more confident when getting frisky. By knowing his sensitive areas, the true range of "normal" penis appearances, and how men experience orgasm, you'll be that much more at ease when you're being intimate. This chapter will do all that, and much more. And we're going to start just south of the border.

HIS PENIS

Between articles in women's magazines, gossip in the ladies' room, and urban legend, it's no surprise that many of us aren't sure what to expect when we unzip his pants—especially for the first time. But there's no point making assumptions based on these massively unreliable sources. You'll only end up feeling even more confused. So let's check out the facts. What *is* the average penis size, anyway? Why do men get erections? What happens if you swallow his semen? We're going to cover all the bases, so let's get going.

EXTERNAL PENIS ANATOMY

Let's start with what's in front of us. What do you see when you look at his package? Here's a quick rundown on what's what.

The penis is the male sex organ, and it becomes erect when stimulated. It's used both for reproduction—for delivering semen into the vagina—and for urination. (Luckily, it's impossible for both of those things to happen at the same time. You'll find out why in a few pages.) The glans is the sensitive head of the penis, filled with nerve endings. That means it's extremely sensitive, and focusing on it during oral sex can be highly arousing for him. The corona is the ridge of the glans, or penis head. The frenulum is the thin fold of skin on the underside of the glans, and it's extra sensitive. If you're giving oral sex, licking or lightly touching the frenulum can add extra pleasure.

If your partner is not circumcised, his penis will sport an additional fold of muscle tissue called the foreskin. It covers and protects the glans. Men who have not been circumcised tend to have higher sensitivity of the glans due to the high concentration of nerves in the foreskin.

The shaft is the body of the penis. When the penis is not erect, the skin on the shaft is loose, leaving room for it to stretch when an erection occurs. The shaft contains three tubes of erectile tissue. Two of the tubes are called the corpora cavernosa, and the third tube is called the corpus spongiosum. This third tube contains the urethra, which transports both urine and semen.

The testicles are the male gonads, and they produce sperm and hormones. They are contained within the scrotum, which is simply a pouch of skin. The scrotum maintains the testicles at a specific temperature to keep sperm alive and healthy. In colder temperatures, the scrotum pulls closer to the body in order to absorb more body heat for the testicles.

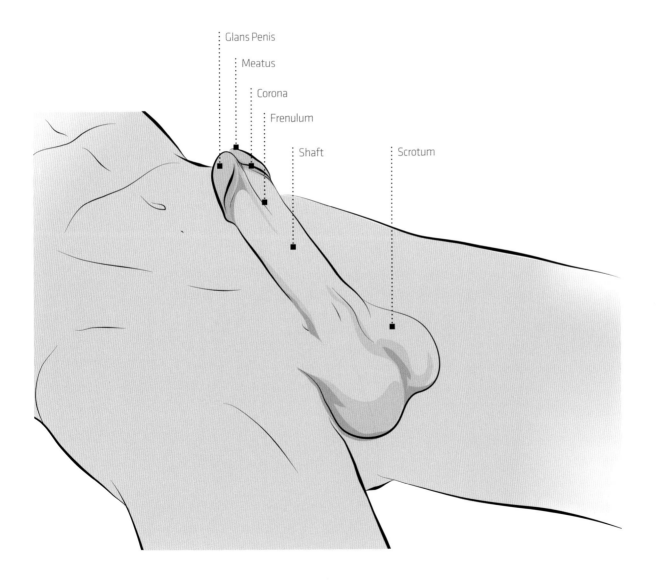

Glans Penis

Meatus

Corona

Frenulum

Shaft

Scrotum

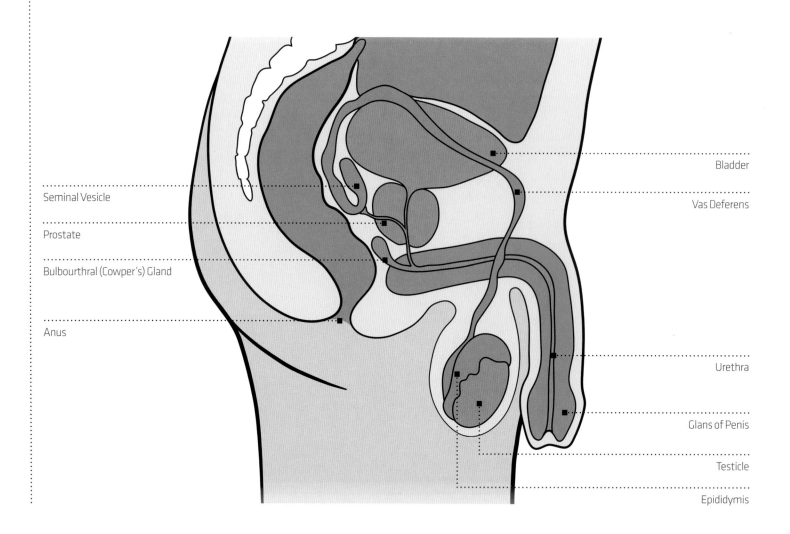

Bladder

Seminal Vesicle

Vas Deferens

Prostate

Bulbourthral (Cowper's) Gland

Anus

Urethra

Glans of Penis

Testicle

Epididymis

INTERNAL PENIS ANATOMY

Now let's take a closer look. What's going on inside the penis? Here's what's invisible to the naked eye …

Within the testicles are coiled tubes called the seminiferous tubules, which produce sperm. The epididymis is the coiled tube at the back of the testicles where the sperm matures. When a man becomes aroused, contractions cause his sperm to move into the vas deferens, which are two ducts. The vas deferens move the mature sperm to the urethra when he's ready to ejaculate. The ejaculatory ducts connect the vas deferens and the seminal vesicles. These ducts empty sperm into the urethra. The urethra stops the flow of urine and transports semen for ejaculation when the time is right.

Seminal vesicles are the glands at the end of each vas deferens, and they secrete a sugar-laden fluid that gives the sperm fuel for movement. The prostate is a gland located beneath the bladder. This walnut-sized gland produces fluid that, combined with the fructose-rich fluid from the seminal vesicle, nourishes the sperm. The prostate is also very sensitive to touch. It is often referred to as the male G-spot or P-spot. You can reach this area directly by inserting your finger into his anus or indirectly by massaging the area between his scrotum and bum hole, often referred to as the taint (as in "it *ain't* his balls and it *ain't* his bum"). The urethra runs through the center of the prostate gland, while the Cowper's glands are pea-sized glands located on each side of the urethra that secrete an alkaline substance called preejaculatory fluid. This fluid coats the urethra to ensure the safe passage of sperm. Sometimes called precum, though its main function isn't carrying sperm, it can have traces of sperm nonetheless, and can therefore cause pregnancy.

PENIS SIZE: IS BIGGER REALLY BETTER?

Penis size is certainly an ego factor for most men, but the reality is, penis size doesn't matter very much when it comes to sex. When erect, the average penis size is 5–6 inches (12.7–15.2 centimeters) in length, and 1.5 inches (3.8 centimeters) in diameter. Occasionally, women complain that sex is painful with men whose penis size is significantly larger than average—but that's pretty rare. Typically, that pain or discomfort results from a lack of lubrication, stress, or starting to have sex before being fully aroused. The vagina is constructed to be able to stretch to accommodate giving birth as well as penis size, so variations in penis size don't necessarily make for painful intercourse.

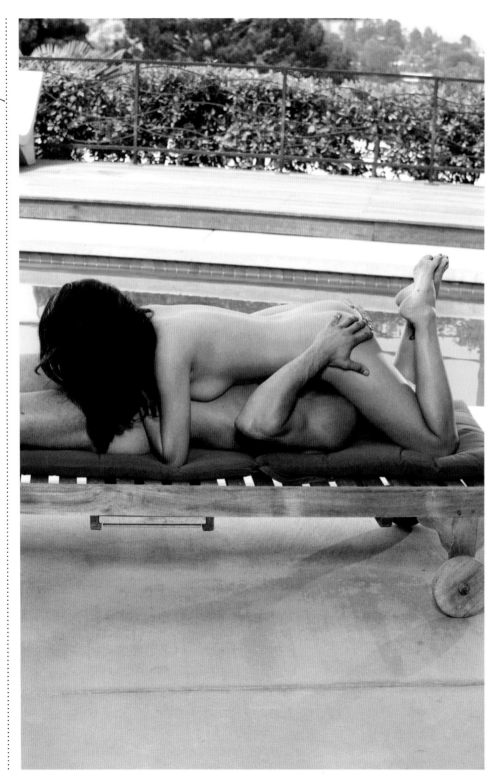

ALL ABOUT SEMEN

What's this mysterious fluid that's projected from your partner's penis—and what are you supposed to do with it? Can he control it? Well, ejaculation is a reflexive act, but men are able to learn how to control the length of time it takes to ejaculate. That involves mastering sexual excitement, which is a psychological process, and controlling the musculature of the penis, which is a physical act. You can support your partner by helping him slow down when he's close to ejaculation; that'll help his erection last longer.

Here's the lowdown on your partner's semen:

How much? On average, anywhere from about half a teaspoon to two teaspoons of semen is released upon ejaculation. During ejaculation, he experiences about ten to fifteen muscle contractions; the second muscle contraction usually releases most of the semen, while the following contractions release smaller amounts.

What's in it? Contrary to popular belief, semen is relatively low in protein, but it's high in sugar. It's also made up of enzymes, amino acids, vitamin C, and zinc. Is it fattening? Nope. The average ejaculation contains about five to twenty calories.

Typically, semen is clear in color, but can also have a white, gray, or yellow tint. Immediately after ejaculation, semen coagulates, or thickens, to help it remain inside the vagina and increase the possibility of fertilization. After a period of fifteen to thirty minutes, the semen liquefies again so that it can swim up the vagina in the hopes of fertilizing an egg.

Can it transmit STIs? Yes. This is really important. Semen can transmit STIs like HIV, herpes, hepatitis B, gonorrhea, and chlamydia. In rare circumstances, it can also contain blood, which carries viruses and other diseases. That's why you shouldn't brush your teeth immediately after giving oral sex, especially if you're with a new partner. Brushing your teeth may cause microtears in your gums, which can increase the likelihood of infection.

Does swallowing matter? Swallowing his semen won't make you any more or less likely to orally contract an STI. If you've given oral sex, at least trace amounts of preejaculatory fluid have already entered your mouth. That means you need to be careful about using protection, even with oral sex.

Spit or swallow? Do you spit or swallow? That seems to be the major question regarding giving oral sex. But when it comes to his cum, you have plenty of other options than just those two. Since swallowing semen doesn't put you at an additional risk of STIs, the deciding factor should be whether you're comfortable with it. If you are, go for it. If not, consider encouraging him to finish on your body. Watching him orgasm can be really exciting because you'll get to witness his physical response to your mutual pleasure. He could ejaculate on your stomach, on your breasts, in your hands—or anywhere else that turns you both on.

If you do choose to have him finish in your mouth, spitting the semen out is always an option. (Be sure to have a towel nearby for just such an event.)

What does it taste like? Well, semen usually has a pretty neutral taste, but that can vary due to lifestyle factors such as diet and stress. Typically, smoking and eating fried or fatty foods are believed to make semen taste worse, while eating fruits and vegetables rich in natural sugars, such as watermelon, pineapples, apples, and fruit juices, make it taste better. If you're worried about the taste of semen or about the sensation of ejaculate in your mouth, keep a towel nearby in case you choose to spit. And be sure to have water, a breath mint, or a piece of chocolate handy in case you want to remove its taste quickly and discreetly.

MALE SEXUAL RESPONSE CYCLE: HOW HE GETS OFF

While it's true that both men and women experience the four stages of sexual response—excitement, plateau, orgasm, and resolution—described by Masters and Johnson, men experience arousal and orgasm differently than women do. Of course, both men and women can enjoy immense pleasure during sex, but the physical, hormonal, and orgasmic experiences that produce that pleasure aren't the same.

When your partner is sexually stimulated, blood flow to his pelvic area will increase, producing an erection. That means he's in the excitement phase. His erection isn't necessarily dependent on how aroused he is, though. Psychological, neurological, and circulatory factors (among others) can influence how hard he gets, and how quickly. As his penis hardens, the diameter of his urethra doubles, his scrotal tissue thickens, and his testicles retract close to his body. His muscles tense, and his blood pressure and heart rate increase.

While he's aroused, your partner is in the plateau phase. If he gets distracted, it's more likely that he will lose his erection during this phase than the excitement phase. As he gets closer to orgasm, the head of his penis will become more swollen, and may become red or purple in color. His testicles double in size and retract further into the body. Preejaculatory fluid, or precum, may be released by the Cowper's gland at this point. His muscle tension increases even more and sometimes results in spasms. You'll know he's approaching orgasm if his toes curl, or if he makes clutching or grasping movements with his hands. He'll be breathing heavily, his heart rate can spike up to 100–175 beats per minutes, and his blood pressure will continue to rise. You'll notice sex flush, or reddening of the skin on his face, neck, and back.

Before your partner orgasms, he'll experience a sensation and instinct that men call "ejaculatory inevitability." That's the beginning of the smooth muscle contractions that lead to orgasm, and it's also when his semen is deposited near the top of the urethra, ready for ejaculation. What does it feel like? Tommy, forty, says, "It feels like what a volcano might feel like: intense pressure. I feel warmth wash over me and I know that an orgasm is about to happen." Once a man reaches this point, he can't pull back from orgasm. Then, when he does orgasm, the muscles around his penis and anus contract in 0.8-second intervals. The first few contractions are the most intense, and release the majority of the semen. Subsequent contractions are less intense, and more spaced out. He'll also experience more involuntary muscle contractions, which result in pelvic thrusting, spasms in the hands and feet, and arching of the spine. His breathing, heart rate, and blood pressure have peaked.

Unlike the female body, the male body returns to its prearousal state right after orgasm. During his resolution phase, half of his erection recedes immediately. The diameter of the urethra returns to its normal size, and the testicles begin to descend from the body. On average, it takes about five minutes for his muscle tension to relax (although total resolution may take as long as two hours). Many men fall asleep soon after orgasm due to the body's rapid return to normal functioning. After climaxing, men experience a refractory period that prevents them from being restimulated to orgasm. The length of this period depends on the individual, and can vary according to his age and his mood. But here's a point of reference: the average man in his late thirties needs about thirty minutes or more before he can be restimulated. Most men feel satisfied with one orgasm per sexual encounter.

MEET THE PENIS: HAND JOB HOW-TO

A hand job—that is, manual stimulation of the penis—is a great way to get to know your partner's penis. Touching, stroking, and caressing his penis can be done for its own pleasure, as part of foreplay, or to reach orgasm. His penis is highly sensitive, so even simple stroking and touching will be pleasurable for your partner. Every man has his own preferences when it comes to pace, sensitivity, and style of touch, just like you have your own personal preferences when it comes to stimulating your clitoris. So be sure to talk to him during the fun. Ask him if he likes what you're doing, and whether he wants you to go faster or slower. This can be really sexy in itself. Talking about what you're doing adds a second level of eroticism to the act.

Here's how to start. You'll need some lubrication (or your own saliva—some men get turned on by seeing and feeling your saliva on their penises, or by watching you spit on your hands for lubrication). Get your partner to lie back and relax. Wrap your hand firmly around his penis, then begin stroking it in an up-and-down motion. Settle into a slow rhythm and use mild pressure. That's pretty much the basic recipe for a hand job.

But there are plenty of variations to the theme. Here are some suggestions for adding some flavor to a hand job. Just remember not to move too quickly from one style of stimulation to another. It's best to stick to one or two variations per session.

Use two hands. The more stimulation, the better. Stack your hands on top of one another on his penis. This ensures that the entire surface area of his penis is covered by your hands. Start by stroking him with the standard up-and-down motion, then get creative by twisting your hands in opposite directions while squeezing the penis as you move up and down—as if you were (very gently!) wringing a towel dry.

Mix it up. Changing hand job techniques during an encounter is a great way to boost his pleasure, and to keep you interested. Let's face it: using a simple up-and-down motion on your guy until he finishes can sometimes leave you feeling bored—and with a very tired hand. Try starting with one hand, and then using two. Vary the speed. Go super slow, then speed things up. Or, spit on your hand for lubrication, then move your hand around his penis in a twisting motion. Be sure to take your time, though. Stick with each change in technique for at least fifteen to thirty seconds.

Switch up the speed and pressure levels as you build his sexual tension.

Stay edgy. Focus on the edge of the penis's head, right where it meets the shaft. This area is highly sensitive, and he'll love it when you run your fingers over and around it.

Stimulate his frenulum. Draw your fingers over the frenulum. That's the thin line of flesh that is on the underside of the head, and it's supersensitive, too. Try rubbing it lightly with your thumb.

Don't forget the testicles. While massaging his shaft with one hand, use the other to stroke, massage, and lightly squeeze his testicles. Try giving them a gentle tug as you squeeze.

Go further south. After giving his testicles a little love, use your index finger to put light pressure on the perineum, the space between his testicles and his anus.

Using both hands, interlock your fingers around his shaft. Place your thumbs on the frenulum. He'll get an extra jolt of pleasure as you stroke his penis up and down.

Palm him. Place your palms on each side of his penis, and lightly rub them back and forth in the same motion you'd use if you were trying to start a fire by rubbing a stick on a piece of wood.

Alter position and point of view. Change the position of your body while your hands are at work. This lets you experiment with different angles, and it also gives him a new visual, which can be really exciting.

Make eye contact. Be sure to make eye contact with him while your hands are pleasuring his penis. That'll up the intimacy and connection. Plus, it'll turn him on even more, because he'll know that you're paying attention to his reactions.

Of course, there are also a few simple don'ts when it comes to hand jobs. First, don't grip him too hard. There's a fine line between a firm grip and a grip of death. Start with a light level of pressure and ask him how it feels as you grip tighter. He'll tell you when the pressure feels right. Second, don't go too fast. Increasing the speed of your strokes as your handiwork progresses can feel good for him, but it's important to start slow. Speed can cause painful friction for him if you're not using enough lubrication. Also, don't focus exclusively on the shaft. It's easy to think of a hand job as simply moving your hand in an up-and-down motion—but, like I've told you, there's so much more to it! Pay attention to his entire package: the head, testicles, and perineum.

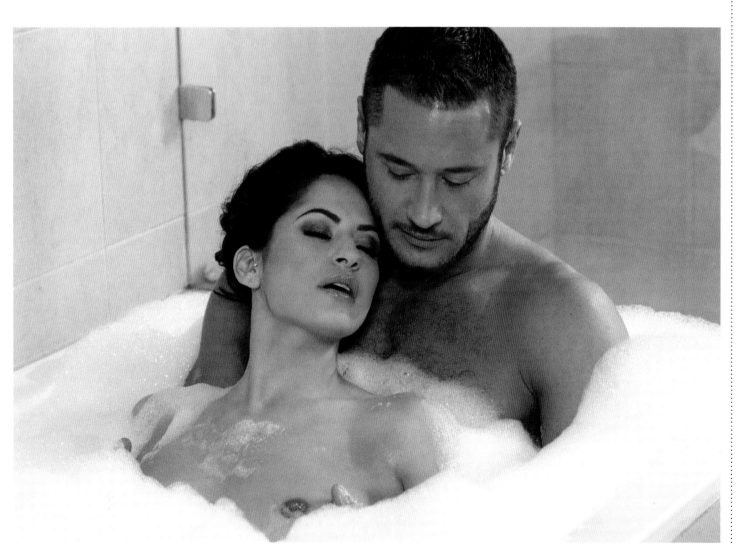

Also, don't look bored. The fact is, it may take a while for your partner to climax, and you might start to feel bored and impatient, and your hands might get tired, too. Try not to let your mind wander to your to-do list at work, or to when you're going to get around to painting that ceiling. Stay in the moment, and do change up your styles and positions. It'll be more fun for you if you can stay engaged, and it'll be more exciting for him if he knows that you're into it. Don't be afraid to speak up. Talk about what's going down, and how exciting it is. Tell him what you love about touching him and be proactive in asking him what he wants you to do. Does technique matter? Yes. But enthusiasm and showing him that you are really into it trumps technique every single time.

PENIS PROBLEMS

Your partner's penis is probably a big part of how he views his masculinity and virility. That means experiencing difficulty with erections—and other physical issues that center on the penis—can be emotionally difficult for both him and you. Following are the most common penis-related problems that men experience, what you need to know about them, and what you can do to help.

ERECTION ISSUES

Erectile dysfunction, or ED, is the inability to achieve or maintain an erection during a sexual interaction, and it can be caused by a number of medical and psychological factors. Regardless of the cause, men who suffer from ED tend to feel depressed or anxious. And it's really common: about 40% of men experience it on at least one occasion. If your partner is having problems with his erection, remember that you are not to blame. Suggest that he see his family doctor, and be sure to tell him that he has your full support, because discussing ED is hard for most men. His physician will determine whether the root of the issue is physical or psychological. Factors such as stress, depression, and lack of confidence can impact his ability to get an erection and reach orgasm. If that's the case for your partner, talk therapy with a licensed psychotherapist may be helpful.

EJACULATION ISSUES

The most common ejaculation problem men experience is premature ejaculation—that is, when a man reaches orgasm after only a short period of stimulation. The *International Classification of Diseases* defines premature ejaculation as reaching orgasm within fifteen seconds of beginning intercourse. About 30% of men have experienced premature ejaculation

on at least one occasion, and it can happen more frequently with age. Like ED, its causes can be either physical or psychological. If it's happening to your partner, ask him to tell you when he feels close to orgasm. Slowing down the sexual encounter, going back to light foreplay, or even distracting him from intercourse can help delay ejaculation. It's very possible for the two of you to work through his ejaculation problems together, so do give him your support, patience, and care.

SEXUALLY TRANSMITTED DISEASES

Sometimes, difficulty getting and maintaining an erection can be the result of an STI. During one study on ED, researchers found that participants who had had an erectile problem were more likely to have had a prior STI and had usually had more than five partners during the previous year. STIs can also lead to a general lack of interest in sex due to physical discomfort, psychological stress, or shame. It's always important to get tested regularly to rule out possible STIs.

EMOTIONAL ISSUES

Emotional concerns can also be responsible for your partner's issues with arousal. In 2011, *The Journal of Sex Research* published the findings from a study on predictors of men's sexual desire. In this study, researchers asked men about psychological adjustment, dysfunctional sexual beliefs, automatic thoughts, emotions during sex, and medical conditions. Their findings showed that relationship satisfaction doesn't have a negative impact on male sexual desire and arousal. The emotional factors that do impact his ability to get it up include restrictive attitudes toward sexuality, lack of erotic thoughts during sex, concerns about getting an erection, and sexual shame (that is, feeling guilty about being sexual). If your partner is struggling with emotional issues such as these, be as positive as possible and encourage him to stay in the moment with you. That may help him relax, get aroused, and stay that way.

MEDICAL TREATMENTS FOR ED

If your partner has been diagnosed with ED, his physician may suggest prescription medication, such as sildenafil, which is also known as Viagra. Viagra is intended to increase his ability to get and maintain an erection, but many couples also assume that it'll improve their relationship satisfaction overall. That's a myth: while men taking Viagra often report higher self-esteem and improved feelings of sexual competency, they reported no overall change in the quality of their relationships. It's likely, though, that your relationship *will* improve through

better communication, or by meeting with a therapist who specializes in couples' therapy and sexuality. While it's certainly important to treat the physical issues that may be causing his difficulties with erection, it's just as important for your partner to be able to voice his frustration and anxiety. Whether you're seeing a therapist together or not, you can help your partner by being empathetic and listening to his concerns.

Remember that Viagra is a prescription drug, and the only way to get it is by seeing your doctor. It's sometimes prescribed to counteract the sexual side effects of some medications, especially psychiatric medications, which can have a negative impact on sexual arousal and response. Due to possible side effects and interactions with other medications, it's really important to consult with a doctor before taking Viagra, or before changing your dosage.

Popular myth suggests that Viagra is a magic bullet when it comes to male arousal. The truth is, it's really not. Here's the science behind Viagra. When your partner is stimulated or aroused, the nervous system in the erectile tissue in his penis releases nitric oxide. That, in turn, stimulates an enzyme that produces a "messenger" compound, which is called cyclic guanosine monophosphate, or cGMP. The cGMP relaxes the smooth muscle

cells in the penis. Then the arteries in the penis dilate, or widen, and the blood flows into the penis more easily. The erectile tissue fills with blood, which results in—you guessed it—an erection. Viagra works by maintaining the level of cGMP in the smooth muscle cells. It's important for your partner to take Viagra about an hour before sex.

Now you're down with the particulars of the penis, and you're an expert when it comes to his sexual response. That means you can give him that much more pleasure next time you get it on—and you can make it your pleasure, too. It's true that men and women experience sex and sexuality differently due to biological and hormonal factors, but at the end of the day, both genders crave pleasure and sexual connection with a partner. Speaking of which, the next chapter will show you how to be mistress of the highest art of sexual connection: seduction. Read on!

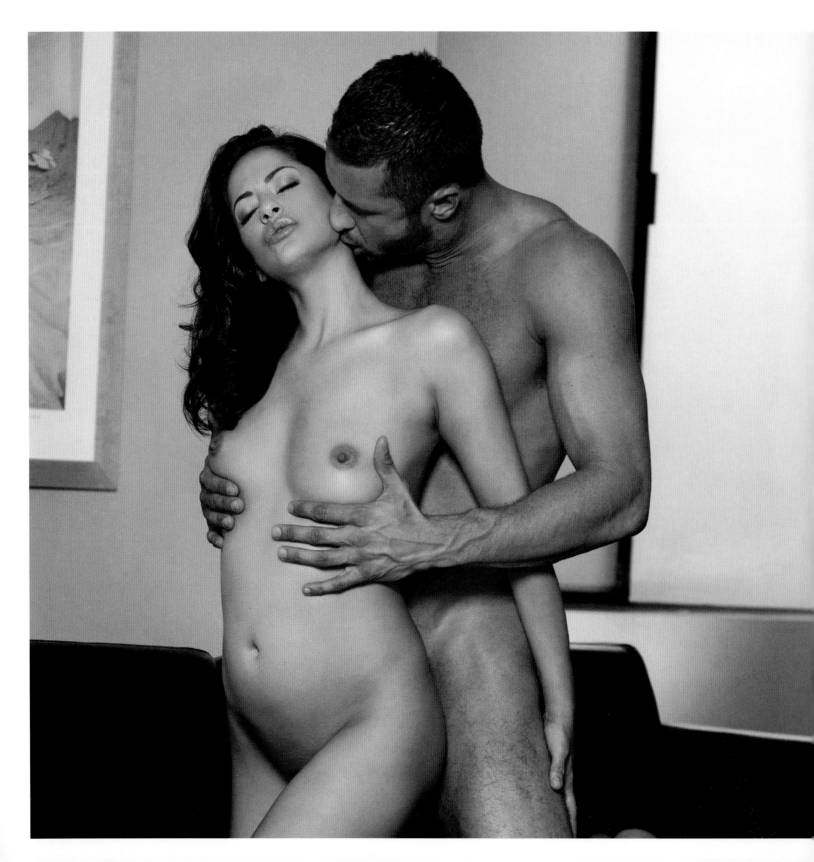

07 *Sex Positions: Poses That Boost Passion and Pleasure*

What are the keys to incredible sex? Connection, passion, and staying in the moment. Beware of the magazines and websites that proclaim that a "new" or "secret" sex position is all you need. There are no such new or secret sex positions—and no one sex position works for all women or couples. All you need to know are the basics, plus a few safe and effective variations. That's why this chapter gives you a breakdown of sex positions, with easy adaptations you can incorporate into your sexual repertoire. Think of this chapter as an inspirational guide, and experiment with the positions that pique your interest. And remember, there's no formula or recipe when it comes to great sex. As long as you're comfortable and aroused, anything goes.

WHY SHOULD YOU KNOW YOUR SEXUAL POSITIONS?

As the saying goes, knowledge is power—and when it comes to your sexuality, knowledge is also empowerment. The more you know, the better off you are, because being aware of your options gives you the ability to choose what's right for you. Being familiar with a range of sexual positions can:

Help you reach orgasm. If you're savvy when it comes to sexual positions, you'll be able to experiment and discover which positions best help you reach the big O.

Add variety and fun to your sex life. When you're able to switch up sex positions, whether it's during the same encounter or over the course of your relationship with your partner, you've got the power to add novelty and variety to your sex life—any time you want to. Just like eating the same thing every day can become monotonous—even if it's a luscious, decadent ice-cream sundae—sex can become routine if you do it the same way all the time. Switch things up: variety is exciting.

Choose your best view. Different sex positions can offer different visual perspectives. For example, being able to see your genitals (or his) while you're having sex can be really stimulating. Watching his facial expressions during sex can add to your excitement: seeing him respond to pleasure can increase your pleasure, too.

Here's an easy-to-follow guide to basic sexual positions. You can add endless variations to these positions: each variation can be new and exciting, and the sexual possibilities are only limited by what works for your bodies. Remember, everyone's body is different and different couples come together differently. Don't believe magazines that promise positions guaranteeing orgasm. While certain positions do hit certain hot spots like the clitoris or the G-spot more effectively—which *can* help you reach orgasm more easily—only you can figure out what your go-to positions are. So go ahead and experiment, and see what works best for you.

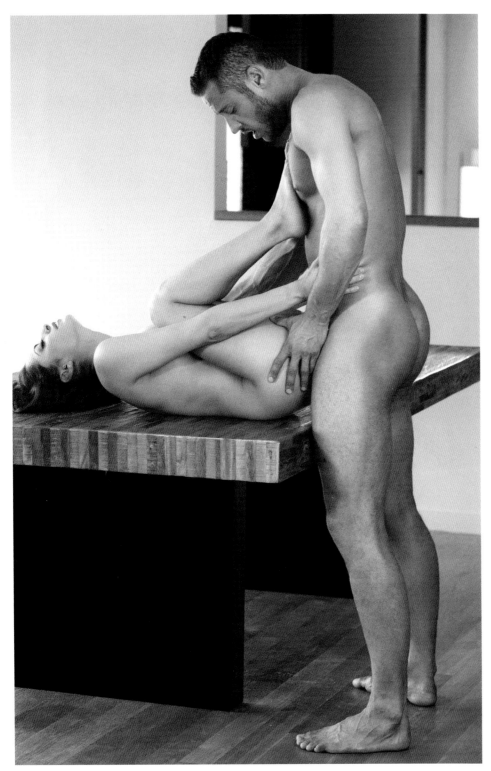

MAN ON TOP (MISSIONARY STYLE)

To start, lie flat on the bed or the floor. Spread your legs and elevate them slightly by either bending your knees and keeping your feet on the bed or floor, or by raising your legs up and off of the bed or floor altogether. Your partner will move between your legs and penetrate you while facing you. You might want to wrap your legs around your partner's waist, or rest them on his shoulders or hips—or anywhere else that's comfortable for both of you.

Benefits

• *Intimacy.* Because you're face to face with your partner, this position is especially intimate. It allows eye contact and a close embrace.

• *Your control.* The missionary position allows your partner to implement thrusting speed and intensity, but you can adjust depth of penetration by thrusting your own hips up.

• *Comfort.* Your pelvic floor muscles are more relaxed in the missionary position, making sex more comfortable—especially if you feel a little nervous.

Challenges

• *Stomach contact.* Since your chest and belly are pressed tightly against your partner's, this position isn't suitable for the later stages of pregnancy.

• *Body size.* Having sex in the missionary position might be more difficult if your partner is heavy or obese.

• *No clitoral contact.* This position is less likely to stimulate the clitoris directly.

Variations and Tips

• *Do it yourself.* To add stimulation while you're in the missionary position, don't be afraid to use your fingers to massage your clitoris. (Plus, while you're giving your clitoris a little attention, the rest of your hand will be able to feel the base of his shaft as it moves in and out of you.)

• *Get flexible.* In the "standard" missionary position, your legs are spread but lie relatively flat on the bed. Try to move your legs higher by bending your knees and placing them on his chest. If you're flexible, rest your calves over his shoulders. This angle will allow for deeper penetration, G-spot stimulation, and more intense thrusting.

• *Have him stand up.* This variation can be really comfortable for both of you. Try having your partner penetrate you while he's standing on the floor; meanwhile, you're lying on the edge of the bed with your legs spread and slightly bent.

• *It's all in his hips.* While the full length of his penis is inside you, have him shift his body upward and then immediately downward, so that his pelvic bone rubs against your pubic mound and clitoris. This move is great for both clitoral stimulation and for feeling the full depth of penetration.

• *The big squeeze.* Wrap your legs around him to hold him closer for maximum body contact. That'll make this position even more intimate than it already is.

• *Use props.* Place a pillow, folded blanket, or foam wedge under your hips to lift them at an angle: this creates better G-spot stimulation (and that can only be a good thing!).

• *Arms and the man.* Get your partner to vary the position of his upper body: he can lie flat on top of you, hold his weight with his elbows, or support himself by pushing straight up with both arms.

WOMAN ON TOP

Have your partner lie flat on his back on the bed or the floor. Kneel beside him, then swing one knee over his body so that you're straddling his hips. Use your hand to hold or stabilize his penis. (Feel free to use a little lubricant or saliva on your hand to masturbate him for a few moments prior to penetration.) Now, slowly lower your body onto his while you guide his penis into your vagina. Use your legs to keep your body stable, and use both legs and hips to take charge of the movement, speed, and direction of the thrusting. Try to use slow, controlled motions to start. Because you're the one doing the "riding" in the Woman on Top, it's also known as the "Cowgirl" position.

Benefits

• *Great for pregnancy.* Since there's no pressure on the stomach in this position, it's easy to enjoy sex in the Woman on Top position when you're pregnant.

• *G-spot friendly.* The position and angle of your body during this position makes it easy for his penis to stimulate your G-spot.

• *You're in control.* When you're on top, you have full control of the speed, intensity, and depth of the penetration.

• *He loves what he sees.* This is a very visual position for your partner, since he has a full view of your face and breasts, and can easily see his penis penetrating you.

• *Hands-free.* In this position, both you and your partner have free hands, so use them. Run your fingers through your hair, caress your breasts, play with your clitoris, and encourage him to touch you as well. Make the most of this great position.

• *He may last longer.* Since your partner has a limited range of motion in the Woman on Top, he might be able to last longer before orgasming—and that means more pleasure for both of you.

Challenges

• *Fatigue.* This position can be especially hard work for your legs. If your thigh muscles start to burn, place your feet under your thighs and push up on them. You can also lean on his chest with one or both hands for stability, or you can stay still while he does the thrusting.

Variations and Tips

• *Reverse Cowgirl.* Get into the Woman on Top position—but mount him backward, so that your back is facing him. From there, you can lean forward and hold on to his legs for stability, or arch your back and place your hands on his chest behind you. The Reverse Cowgirl offers you a different angle and range of motion from the standard Woman on Top position—and he'll love the visuals in this position, since seeing your butt moving up and down on his pelvis will be incredibly arousing for him.

• *Circle and grind.* While your hips are pressed all the way down on his pelvis, move your hips in a circle and grind them into his pelvic bone. Performing these motions simultaneously can help you reach a blended orgasm.

• *Be a tease.* Since you're in full control of penetration in this position, why not tease him a bit before he penetrates you fully? Grab his penis at the base and rub it against your vulva. Or press his penis laterally against your vulva and move your hips up and down against his shaft. Then, when you're ready, insert only the head, or tip, of his penis into your vagina. Move up and down slowly—and when you're ready, take the full length of his shaft inside of you.

• *Relax a little.* You're on top, but that doesn't mean you have to do all the work. Take some of the pressure off by leaning forward. At the same time, have him bend his knees. This creates leverage to help him thrust into you while your body is stationary.

• *Do it sideways.* Try the lateral coital position, recommended by well-known sex researchers Masters and Johnson. This position is similar to the traditional Woman on Top position, except that the woman shifts her weight to her right side. While you're in the Woman on Top position, get him to grab your bent left knee while his right knee is bent to increase stability. Then, you shift your weight to your right side while straightening your right leg. This position lets both you and your partner move freely—neither one of you will feel pinned down. Seventy-five percent of the couples who tried this position in Masters and Johnson's research reported that they preferred it to any other position.

REAR ENTRY

Get on your hands and knees on your bed or the floor. Arch your backside up, so that your partner has easier access to your vagina. Spread your knees about shoulder-width apart and have your partner penetrate you from behind. He can hold your waist or buttocks for support and stability. In this position, the movement or "thrusting" can be done by you, him, or both of you simultaneously.

Benefits

• *Hits the G-spot.* With the Rear Entry position, the penis can penetrate deeper into the vagina for more intense sex and greater G-spot stimulation.
• *Pregnancy-friendly.* Like the Woman on Top position, the Rear Entry can work well if you're pregnant, since it doesn't apply any weight or pressure to your abdomen.

Challenges

• *Depth.* Because this position allows a greater depth of penetration, you may find it difficult, especially the first time you try. Make sure you go slowly and have lubricant on hand in case you find this position challenging.

• *No clitoral contact.* There's no direct clitoral stimulation in the Rear Entry position, so increase your pleasure by using your hands to rub your clitoris. Or encourage your partner to multitask: get him to stimulate you with his free hand.
• *Less intimate.* You're facing away from your partner in this position, which means it might not feel as intimate as the positions in which you're face to face. To bring back the intimacy, straighten your body upright as much as you can, then turn your head and kiss him.

Variations and Tips

• *Change the angle.* Instead of keeping your arms straight, change the angle of his penetration by resting on your elbows. That'll provide you with more overall stability and will place less pressure on your wrists.
• *Achieve lift-off.* While he's inside you, lift your arms off the bed or floor, and, with your back arched, reach up and back to grab his shoulder. This creates a new position in which both of you are kneeling as he enters you from behind.
• *Lie on your belly.* Once he's all the way inside

you, try lying flat on your stomach with your legs together while he lies on his back and penetrates you from above. This "compression" position will make your vagina feel tighter and will place a pleasurable pressure on his penis. To make this variation more comfortable for you, place a pillow under your hips.
• *Standing Rear Entry.* In this variation on the Rear Entry, both partners stand upright. Be sure to face a wall or other solid surface for stability, and arch your back so that he can enter you from behind. Push off the wall to thrust yourself into his hips.
• *Spooning.* The "spoons" position is a side-by-side Rear Entry position. In it, both you and your partner lie side by side, facing the same direction. Even though you're not face to face with your partner, some couples report that they find it just as intimate as cuddling or a close embrace. Plus, this position gives you a free hand to use for manual clitoral stimulation—and allows your partner to caress your breasts and stomach as you have sex. This gentle variation on Rear Entry doesn't place pressure on the stomach, so it's great for pregnancy sex.

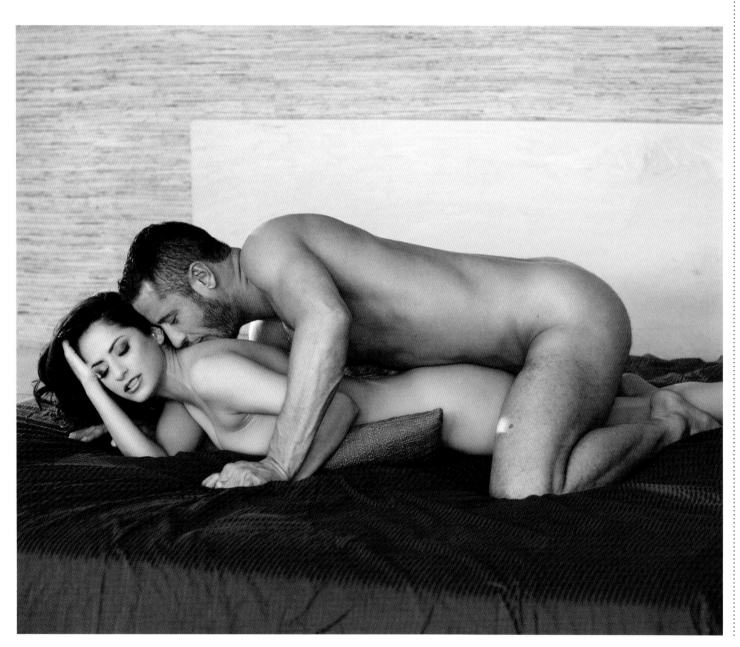

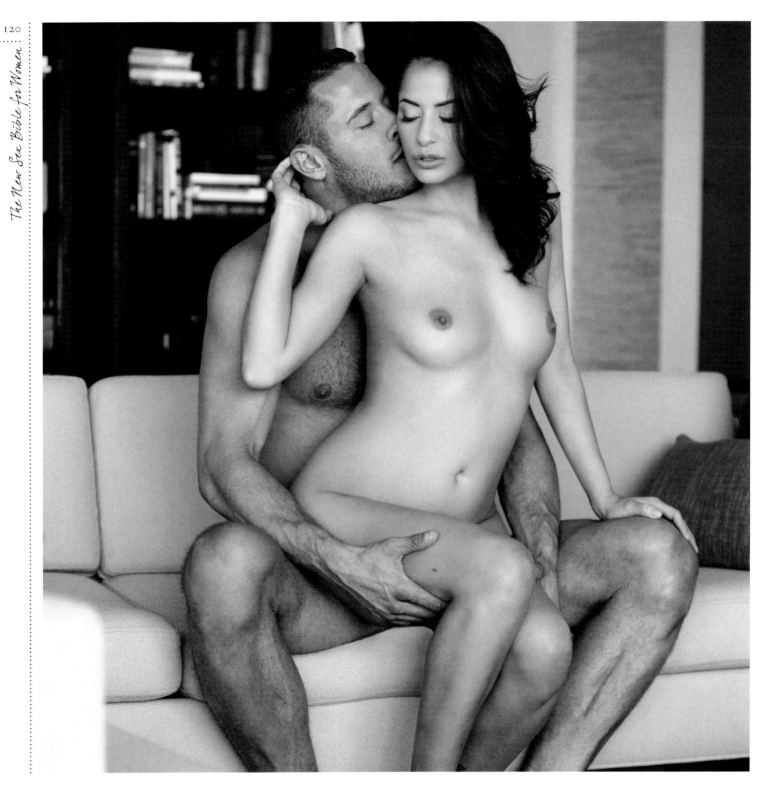

SITTING

Have your partner sit on the bed or the floor, either with his legs straight in front of him or crossed Indian-style. While you're facing him, sit on his lap and wrap your legs around his body. Let him penetrate you and, using your legs, pull your body closer to his until he's fully inside you. Your partner can hold on to your waist or buttocks for support and pull you back and forth toward him as you have sex.

Benefits

• *Intense intimacy.* Because you're facing one another and because your bodies are in almost full contact, this position can really feel intimate. During sex, it's easy to engage in connective eye contact and close embraces.

Challenges

• *It's strenuous.* The Sitting position does require you to do more of the physical work, which may get tiring after a while.
• *Clitoral stimulation.* It's not easy to stimulate your clitoris in this position: it's hard for both of you to reach.

Variations and Tips

• *Circle your hips.* When your partner is fully inside you and when your legs are wrapped tightly around his body, grind your pelvis into his in a circular motion. This circle-and-grind combination is great for both G-spot and clitoral stimulation.
• *Take it to the edge.* Have your partner sit on the edge of the bed with his feet on the floor. Sit on his lap and wrap your legs around him—or sit on his lap facing away from him, with your legs on each side of his hips, in a Reverse Woman on Top position. When he's sitting on the edge of the bed, there's more open space in his lap, making it easier for him to penetrate you.

FIVE ADVANCED POSITIONS FOR INNOVATIVE LOVERS

If you've mastered the basic positions and all of their variations, it may be time to get even more creative. Try these five advanced techniques that require slightly more skill, agility, and balance.

THE PINWHEEL

While you're in the Woman on Top position, get him to lift his back off the bed or floor for a moment, so that you can wrap your legs around his torso. Stretch your arms out behind you to support your body weight. Have him bend his knees, and place one bent leg over your belly while the other leg is under your back. From here, he can place his hands on your thighs to pull you in closer as he thrusts.

Benefits

• *Face to face.* In the Pinwheel, both partners are facing each other, which increases intimacy and lets you see each other's facial expressions—and upper bodies—as you enjoy the encounter.
• *Plenty of support.* Because you're supporting your own body weight with your arms, this is a comfortable position for you: you'll feel stable, not wobbly or off-balance.
• *Pregnancy-friendly.* Try the Pinwheel if you're pregnant. Since there's plenty of support for your body weight and no pressure on your abdomen, it's likely to work well for you.
• *You're in charge.* You direct the angle and depth of penetration in this position, so it's easy to control the level of thrusting to make it comfortable for you.

Challenges

• *It's complicated.* The Pinwheel is a bit more complex than other sitting sex positions—but don't let that put you off! You'll get the hang of it quickly.

Variations and Tips

• *Use those hips.* Since you have control over the movement of your hips in this position, try moving your hips in a circle: it'll make for deeper penetration and increased G-spot stimulation.
• *Give yourself a hand.* The Pinwheel gives you easy access to your clitoris, so take advantage of that. Show him how you love yourself, and play with your clitoris during sex. (He'll have a great view of it in this position.)

THE PEEPSHOW

Lie on your back on the bed or the floor. Have your partner kneel straight up on his knees in front of you. Get him to grab your legs and pull your body upward so that only your shoulders and head are still on the bed (with pillow support for your shoulders, if necessary). Your backside will be in line with his hips, while your knees will be pressed down toward your face, as if you were in the "bicycle" calisthenics position. Hold on to his thighs, if you need to. After he's penetrated you, spread your knees far apart—that'll give him a sexy visual of the action.

Benefits

• *Nice view.* This position allows for exciting visuals. He gets to watch his penis move in and out of you, while you can watch it plunge into you from below.

• *Skip the gym!* While the Peepshow does require agility and strength, it can also help you build up your strength and balance.

Challenges

• *Pressure on shoulders and head.* Because your body weight is resting on your shoulders and head in this position, the Peepshow may be more challenging for women who aren't physically fit. If you feel that your fitness level could use some work, be sure to start slowly and check in with your partner to let him know how you're doing, or if you need to stop.

• *He's in charge.* Since he's in full control of the speed and intensity of penetration in this position, you'll really need to trust that your partner will be mindful of your needs.

Variations and Tips

• *Stay balanced.* Your partner can help keep you steady by holding your ankles. You can also wrap your legs around his waist, or rest them on his shoulders.

• *Touch is key.* Once you feel balanced and stable, try using a free hand to touch yourself, caress his body, or even massage his testicles.

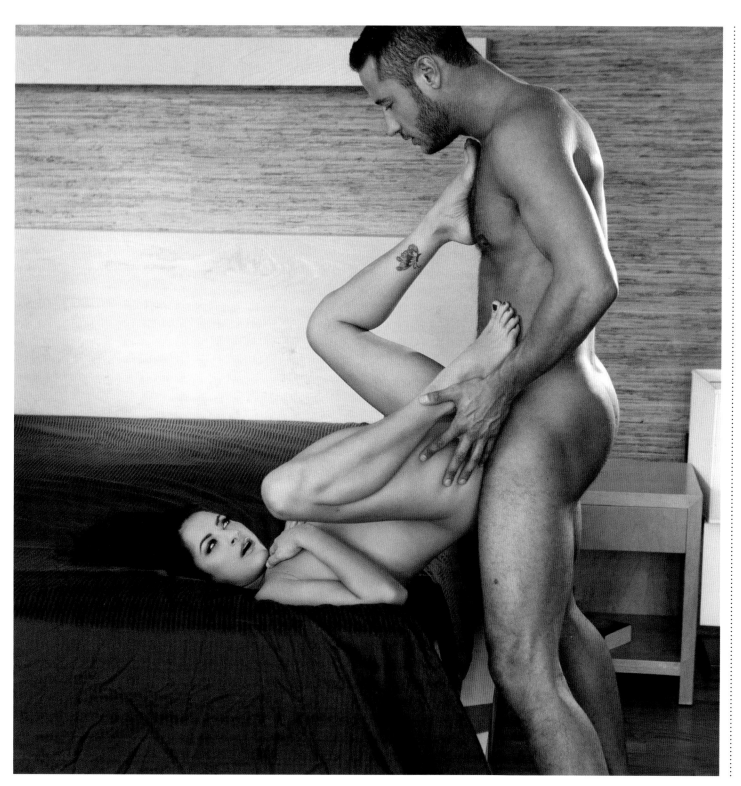

HANDSTAND REAR ENTRY

Have your partner stand behind you: both of you should be facing the same direction. Place your hands on the ground in front of you and let your partner slowly lift your legs (as if you were a wheelbarrow) and penetrate you from behind. This position requires you to have significant arm and upper-body strength.

Benefits

• *Builds muscle.* The Handstand Rear Entry position is nothing if not a strength-builder. It's a fabulous way to build muscle in your arms, shoulders, and abs, and increase your core strength.

• *Feels wild.* This is a fun, exciting take on the standard Rear Entry position—you'll feel sexy and uninhibited in this unusual position.

Challenges

• *Strength level.* The Handstand Rear Entry requires you to have enough upper-body strength to support your full body weight, and to manage to stay balanced while he's thrusting. So proceed with caution! If you're not sure that you're strong enough, build the necessary muscles by doing handstands against a wall at home.

• *No hands.* Since your hands have to remain firmly on the ground in this position, you won't have a free hand to touch yourself or your partner. That means no direct clitoral stimulation.

• *Short-term only.* Your body is at a decline in this position, which means that blood can rush to your head (and away from your genitals). That's why you shouldn't maintain this position for more than a few minutes at a time: don't try to keep it up for the entire encounter.

Variations and Tips

• *Support yourself.* Try lying on the bed and propping yourself up with your arms so that your body is at less of a slope, and to provide comfortable support for your upper body.

THE THIGH MASTER

The Thigh Master is, essentially, a variation of the Reverse Cowgirl position. Get into the Reverse Cowgirl position (see page 117), and, instead of straddling his body with both your legs, place one of your legs between his. Have him raise the knee that's between your legs so that your stomach is close to his thigh. As you ride him, grind your pelvis against his thigh for an extra dash of clitoral pleasure.

Benefits

• *Best of both worlds.* With the Thigh Master, you're on top and are in control of your movements—plus, the position of his thigh lets you stimulate your clitoris while leaving your hands free to caress him, or to hold on to his knee for balance.

• *Set the pace.* As with all Woman on Top positions, being on top allows you to control the speed and intensity of the encounter.

• *Leverage.* It's pretty easy to keep your body stable in the Thigh Master, since you can place your hands on his knees to steady and balance yourself. That means this position may be less tiring than other Woman on Top versions.

• *Pregnancy-friendly.* This position is great for expectant mothers, since it applies no pressure to the abdominal area. You can rest your stomach against his thigh if you like, or you can give your belly a little space by having him lower his knee.

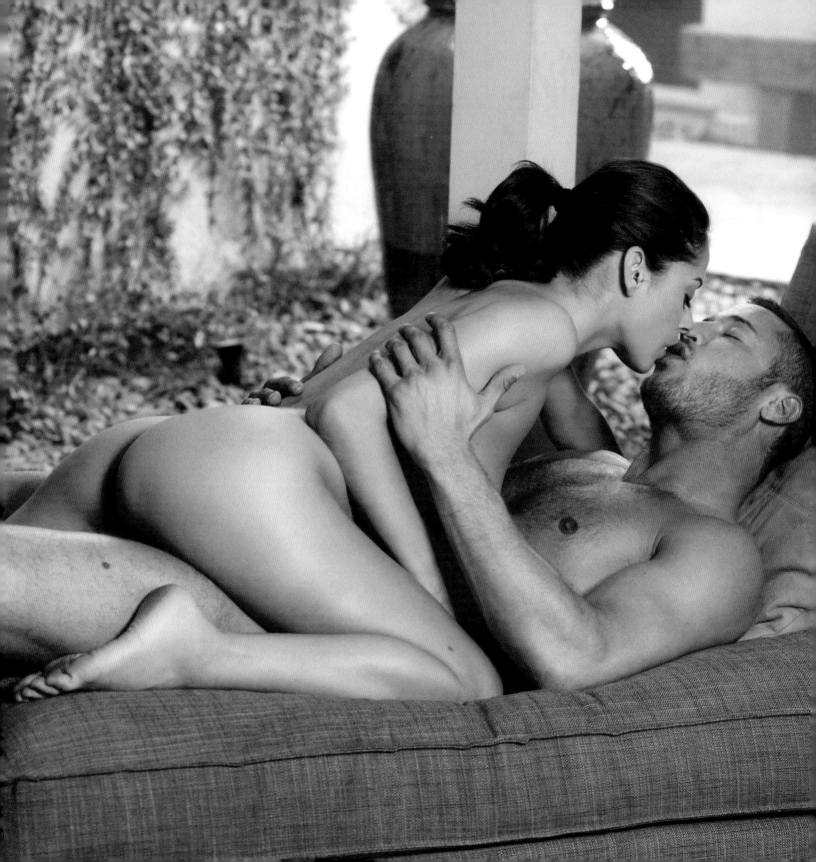

Challenges

• *Fatigue.* Just like any position in which you're on top, you're doing the bulk of the work, so take your time. If you get tired, let more of your body weight rest on your partner, and let him take over by thrusting upward into you.

Variations and Tips

• *Bump, then grind.* You can ride him up and down when you're in the Thigh Master, but you can also circle your hips and grind into his pelvis and thigh for deeper penetration and even more clitoral action.

• *Focus on your clitoris.* Since this position is so clitoris-friendly, be sure to take advantage of it: rub your clitoris against his thigh for some delicious friction.

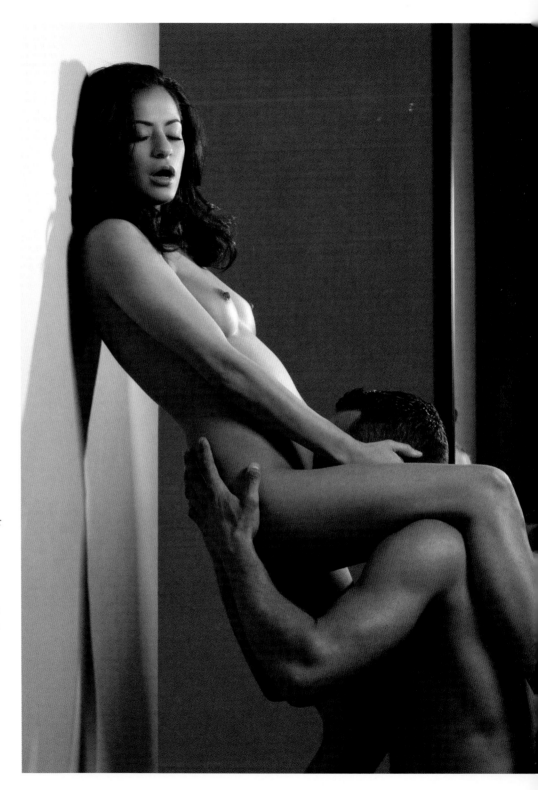

PICK-ME-UP

This position works best if your partner has
a good deal of strength and stamina. While
standing, face your partner and have him pick
you up into his arms. Wrap your legs around his
waist while he supports your body weight with
his arms. He'll move your body up and down as
he thrusts into you. To make it a bit easier for both
of you, have him prop you against a wall.

Benefits
• *No bed necessary.* The Pick-Me-Up is fun and
intense, and having sex away from the "norm"
of the bed can be a really arousing and naughty
change of pace.

Challenges
• *Acrobatics.* This position always looks like it's
so easy to do when you see it in the movies—but
beware. The fact is, to pull it off, your partner
needs to be quite strong, and you really need to
trust him. If those conditions aren't met, the Pick-
Me-Up can be difficult and awkward to achieve.
• *Don't add water.* Because it's important to use
caution with this position, don't attempt it in the
shower: you're likely to slip and hurt yourselves.

Variations and Tips
• *Hit the wall.* If he has a hard time balancing
you in his arms, have him press your back against
a wall.
• *Hold on tight.* Be sure to wrap your
legs around him and hold on to his torso for
stability and safety. Now's the time to use
those thigh muscles!

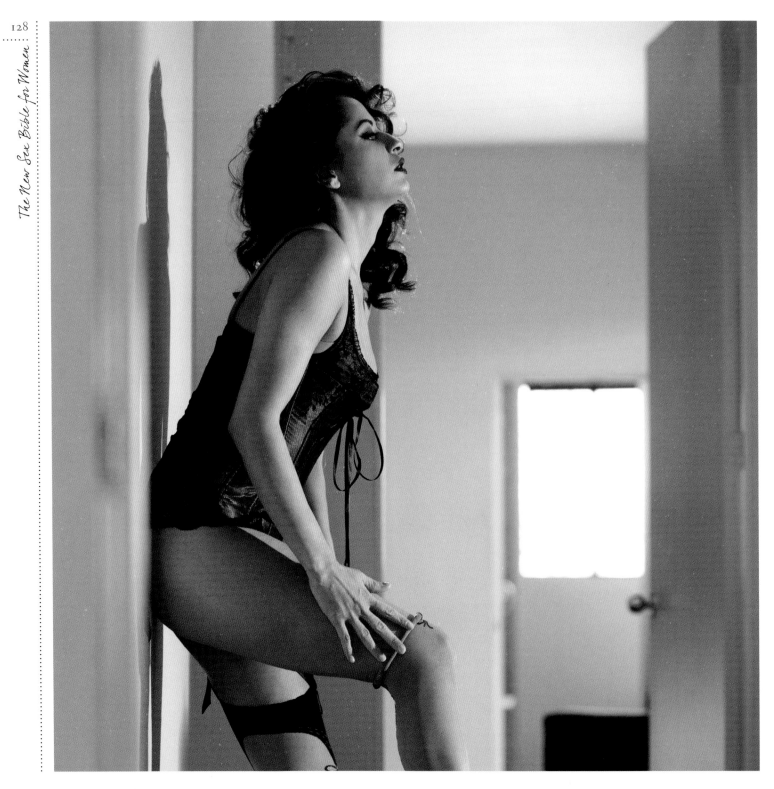

LOCATION, LOCATION, LOCATION

There's no reason to confine sex to the bedroom. In the same way that it's fun to mix things up when it comes to sex positions, you can spice things up by adding variation to *where* you do it. Plus, when you change locations, you'll discover new sex positions without even trying. That'll happen naturally as you make use of your new surroundings. So, why not get creative with the available space in your home? Here are some suggestions for great places to get it on.

BED

The biggest advantage to sex in bed is comfort. A good, springy mattress provides plenty of support for most sex positions. The bed is the best option if you have back or knee problems or issues with balance and mobility. It's also convenient. After orgasm, you can pull up the covers and switch into cuddle mode—or fall right asleep. No need to drag yourself to bed when you're already in it!

Challenges

• *Routine.* Beds are the most common place to have sex—which means they may get a little boring after a while. If you want to keep your bedroom sexy and conducive for hooking up, take out TVs, phones, and other electronic devices, which can be distracting.

Best Positions

• *Half-and-half.* Try having sex while the top half of your body is unsupported by the bed. While you're in the missionary position, let your shoulders and head hang off the side of the bed: the blood that rushes to your head may make your orgasm more intense. Plus, the fact that this position offers less visual stimulation will force you to focus on how your body feels.

• *Rear entry.* Next time you're having sex in the Rear Entry position, have your partner bend you over the bed while you use your knees to brace yourself against it. That'll help keep your body stable during sex.

SHOWER

The shower can be a super-sensual way to get it on. The feeling of warm water cascading over your naked body—and your partner's—can be erotic and relaxing, and adds another layer of sensation to the experience. There's also no better place for foreplay—or for simply caring for each other's bodies—than the shower. Try washing each other slowly and sensually, or give each other long, erotic massages. Use the shower head to explore the way the water pressure feels on your vulva, clitoris, and nipples. (Just don't spray water directly into the vagina because that can lead to an air embolism.) You could also indulge in some oral sex.

Challenges

• *Slippery when wet.* It sounds obvious, but it's easy to forget in the heat of the moment that your bath or shower can get slippery, so be mindful of your safety during shower sex. Make sure you're on firm ground by using a nonslip shower mat. And try not to change sex positions too quickly to avoid losing your balance.

• *Got lube?* Your natural vaginal lubrication will wash away in the shower. If that steamy round of shower sex is going to last more than a few minutes, be prepared: have a silicone-based lubricant on hand to keep the action going.

• *Showers don't love condoms.* If condoms are your choice of protection, shower sex may not be for you. Condoms have not been tested or approved for use in hot, wet environments. But don't let that put you off. Enjoy foreplay in the shower, then head to dry land before putting on the condom.

Best Positions

• *Standing Rear Entry.* This one's great for the bath or shower. Bend over and grab the rim of the tub, a rail, or another secure surface, and have him penetrate you from behind. Go slow to start so you don't slip.

• *Woman on Top.* If you have a bathtub, have your partner lie down in it, then mount and ride him in the Woman on Top or Reverse Cowgirl position.

• *Facing each other.* While you're facing your partner, have him lift your left leg up and place his right hand on your right hip to help stabilize you. Have him penetrate you from the front while standing, and lean back just a little bit in order to get the angle just right. (When you lean back, though, make sure it's against a wall! Always use a nonslip shower mat, and if you need to hold on to something, press your hand against a stable wall, or grip a solid shower handle or towel bar.)

• *Keep it clean.* Make sure the bathroom is clean (nothing is less of a turn-on than hair stuck in the shower drain or soap scum in the tub!) and use soft lighting. Place lit candles around the bathroom to set the mood.

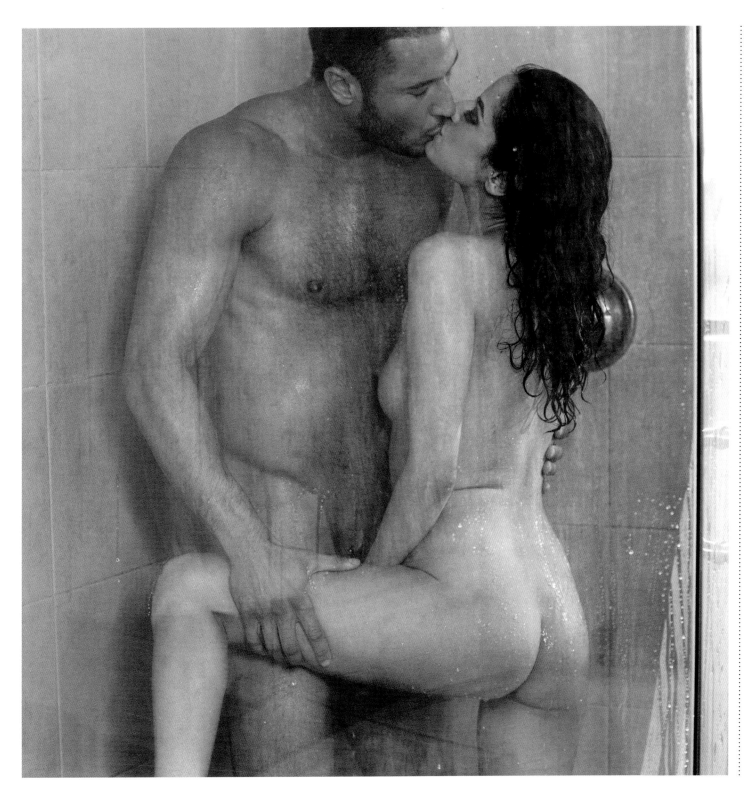

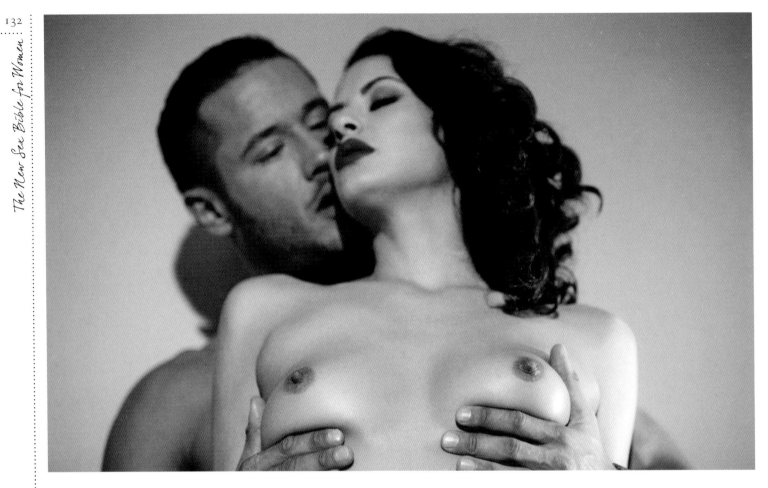

CHAIR OR COUCH

A chair or couch is one of your best bets for stability, which makes it great if you or your partner have injuries or balance and mobility issues. With your partner seated, you can use multiple parts of your body for leverage and stability, which can help you hit hot spots like the clitoris more easily. If you're on top, facing him allows you to grind your hips into him for clitoral stimulation; if you're facing away from him, use your free hand to rub your clitoris. Couches are second only to the bed when it comes to the most comfortable places for sex. It's easy to curl up with each other and cuddle or doze afterward, too. They're a great option for connective sex while not being quite as vanilla as bedroom sex.

Challenges

• *Choose wisely.* Be sure to choose a comfortable chair or couch. A hard wooden dining room chair can be painful when the sex gets more intense.

• *Slippage.* Be careful to choose a chair that isn't going to fall over with two people in it—and see that it isn't on a slippery floor or an area rug.

Best Positions

• *Give him a lap dance.* Get your partner to sit down on a chair or the couch. Moving slowly, you'll walk (or crawl) to him. Then move your hips and body slowly and rhythmically in front of him and near him, hovering over his body and teasing him by rubbing your breasts against him or by lightly kissing or licking him. Face him as you straddle him, and slowly lower yourself onto his penis.

• *Reverse Cowgirl.* While your partner is seated, sit on his lap facing away from him and lower yourself onto his lap. It's a comfortable position for you both, and he'll love the view of your backside moving up and down over him.

• *Rear Entry.* While standing, face a chair so that the seat is pointed toward you. Place one knee on the chair, hang on to the chair's back, then push your backside toward your partner, who will penetrate you from behind.

IN THE CAR

A hot and steamy encounter in a parked car is so exciting: the idea of being caught can be a huge turn-on. It's also perfect for a quickie. Just like sex in the shower, sex in the car is often uninhibited and intense. It might not be that comfortable—but who cares? The two of you will be so aroused, you'll hardly notice.

Challenges

• *Legal issues.* If you're getting it on in a car that's parked anywhere other than your garage, you could be breaking the law—so proceed with caution.

Best Positions

• *Backseat driver.* If you're in the backseat, either Woman on Top or Man on Top works really well. Be sure to push the front seats up as far as they can go so that you have more room to move around.

• *Shotgun.* In the front passenger seat, the easiest position is Woman on Top. You can face him and hold on to the headrest for leverage, or face away from him and grasp the dashboard or windshield.

• *Come prepared.* Be sure to have tissues, a towel, or wet wipes in the car for easy cleanup after he orgasms.

Now it's your turn! The positions I've described in this chapter are just the tip of the iceberg: there's really no limit to the positions you can try. You may be surprised by what comes naturally in the heat of the moment, so start experimenting. Trying new positions adds variety and excitement to your sexual menu—and it's a great way to bring you and your partner closer together. Just be aware of your safety: watch out for wobbly or slippery surfaces so that you don't fall, and if you're not sure of your limits in terms of strength or flexibility, start slow. Talk about each position with your partner afterward—and, most important, have fun.

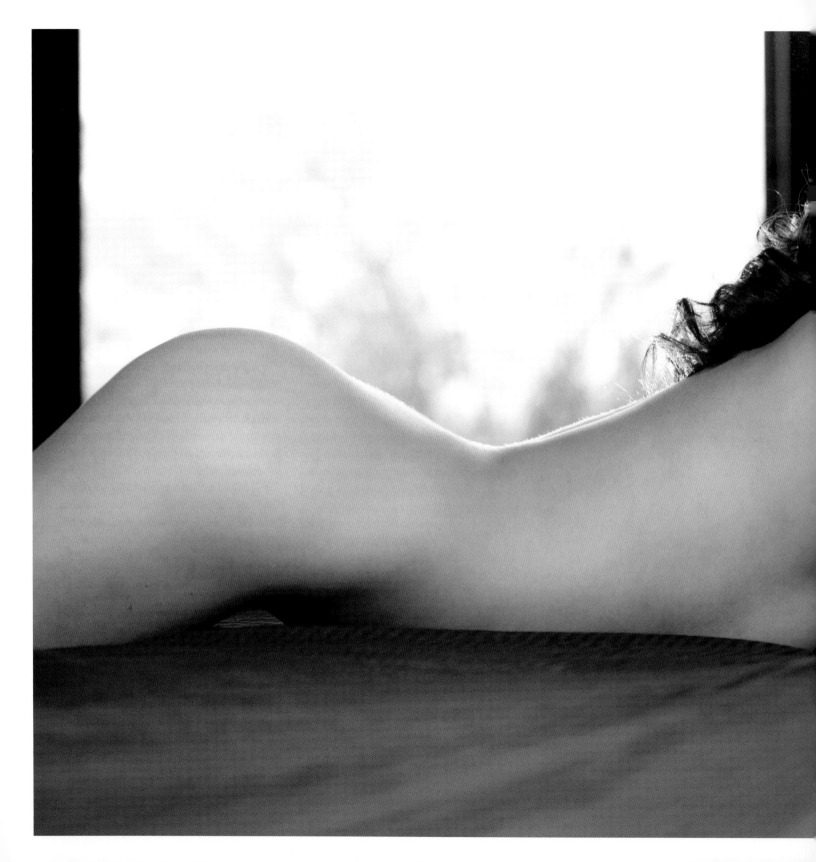

08

Anal Sex: The Forbidden Fruit

For some of us, it's exciting and naughty; for others, it's a complete no-go area. Whichever side of the fence you're on, anal sex is nothing new. In fact, it's very old indeed: ancient art and literature from countries around the globe, such as China, Japan, Greece, and Peru, depict both heterosexual and homosexual anal sex.

While anal sex was considered to be taboo in most Western cultures until recently, its popularity is on the rise today. How do we know? Well, for one thing, anal sex is depicted in adult films more frequently than ever before; it's become almost mainstream, while in the past, it was portrayed as a "niche" or alternative sex act. What's more, surveys from the Centers for Disease Control and Prevention indicated an increase in the reported prevalence of anal sex in both men and women from 1992 to 2005, from 20% to 35% of the United States' sexually active population. (That's an increase of 75%.) And what's caused it? Is the rise in the depiction of anal sex in adult films responsible for it—or, conversely, is it being shown more frequently because the population is engaging in it more often?

I'm not sure what the answer is, but either way, I do know you need to be careful about taking your cues from porn or adult films when it comes to anal sex. It's often represented as common and casual, which can lead viewers to think that anal sex can be spontaneous and careless. The truth is, anal sex requires preparation, communication, and being knowledgeable about your body and about the sex act itself. If you choose to experiment with or regularly engage in anal sex, you need to know how to do it safely, and you need to be aware of the risks. (For example, anal sex doesn't prevent pregnancy, since there is the chance that semen from the anus will find its way into the vagina—an unlikely possibility, but a possibility nonetheless.) For most women, anal play can be pleasurable when it's done with care and caution—so read on to find out how to prepare for anal sex, the best positions for it, how to try it on your partner, and lots more.

WHY ANAL CAN FEEL GOOD

Thanks to the female anatomy, there are two reasons that anal sex might be pleasurable for you. First, the anus contains a large number of nerve endings, making it an erogenous zone. Thus, anything from a feartherlight touch to anal penetration can feel great—if it's done properly and safely. Plus, the internal and external sphincter muscles that are responsible for opening and closing the anus are also membranes that yield both pain and pleasure during anal sex. Second, while the head of the clitoris is visible just above the urethra, it doesn't stop there. The clitoris also extends inside your body, creating a horseshoe shape around the vagina and reaching toward the anus. When you're aroused, both the internal and the external parts of the clitoris fill with blood—just like the penis—and become extremely sensitive.

Aside from the physical pleasures it can offer, anal sex can also be attractive from a psychological perspective. When a taboo surrounds a sexual practice, it often serves to make that practice seem *more* desirable and arousing, not less. While anal sex has a history that spans thousands of years, it's also been forbidden in some cultures—so it's gotten a reputation as being especially naughty. And we all know there's a fine line between naughty and nice that can be particularly erotic. Then there's the fact that anal sex is not directly related to procreation, and is therefore performed purely for sexual gratification rather than conception. Due to the delicate nature of the tissue in the anus and the sex act's former taboo status, engaging in anal sex is often regarded as special or rare. For couples in committed, long-term relationships, anal is sometimes seen as a "gift," or as a type of sex that's reserved for a special occasion.

BASIC ANAL PLAY

Anal intercourse is actually the least common type of anal play. More often, a partner will use his or her finger or mouth, or a sex toy, on the anal area. The following suggestions will help you ease yourself toward anal play before you make the leap to intercourse.

Over the clothes. Have your partner use a finger or two to put pressure on your anal area over your panties or clothing. Be mindful of the sensations that can arise from just this light touch. There's no risk of penetration, so you're less likely to tense up and more likely to pay attention to the pleasure.

Nonpenetrative finger play. Get naked, then have your partner massage your buttocks and surrounding areas—like your hips and thighs—in addition to tracing your anal area with his fingers. Talk to each other and agree that penetration won't happen this time—just light, external touch and massage.

External mouth play. Ask your partner to start by kissing and caressing your buttocks before moving slowly toward your anal area. Agree beforehand that penetration isn't part of the plan, and that he'll only use his fingers and tongue around your anal area. If your partner is going to be licking your anal area, it's highly recommended that he use a dental dam, which is a thin piece of plastic that protects him from unwanted bacteria while still letting you feel all the sensations.

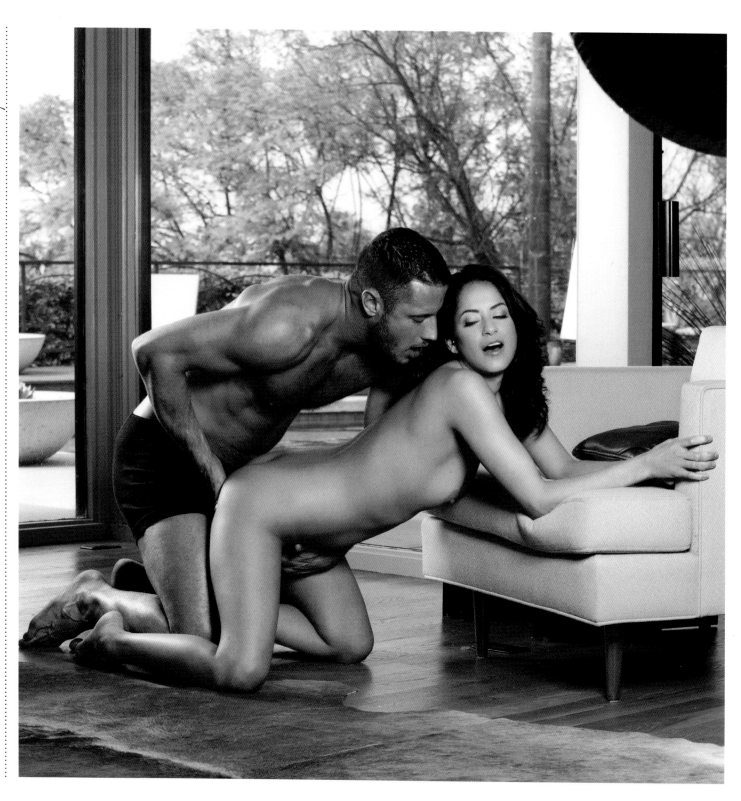

Light penetration. Because even the external anal area has a high concentration of nerves, very small amounts of penetration can be very, very pleasurable. If he's using his tongue to penetrate you, be aware of the potential risk of spreading bacteria and consider using a dental dam (see page 147 for more about these risks). If he's using a finger, be sure to have some lubricant on hand so that it can slide in easily and comfortably. If you are indulging in penetration, lube is essential—so don't skip it. Ever. Unlike the vagina, the anus is not self-lubricating so you'll need to have lube on hand. Aside from making penetration more comfortable, the slipperiness of lube prevents drag and snag on delicate tissues, which could lead to small tears. Use lube for comfort and safety. Lube, lube again, and repeat.

Ask your partner to start slow. Have him begin with external pressure and massage, and slowly transition to gentle penetration with his finger. Get him to insert his finger into your anus up to its second knuckle. Next, have him keep his finger in place, and, when you feel comfortable, ask him to remove it slowly. Repeat the process once or twice, if you can. Keep checking in with him verbally: tell him how you're feeling, and ask him how it feels for him.

Toys. After you become comfortable with gentle anal play and light penetration, it may be time to experiment with toys that are expressly made for use in anal play. Small vibrators can help you relax into anal contact, and can also help relax the muscles around the anus. You can also try anal beads, dildos, and butt plugs (see chapter 10 for a complete rundown on accoutrements for anal enjoyment).

HOW TO PREPARE FOR ANAL SEX

Have a bowel movement. Use the bathroom before engaging in anal sex or anal play. A healthy person will be able to rid his or her bowels of most fecal matter with a single trip to the bathroom, but there may still be traces of feces in the anus. The fact is, the more you engage in anal play, the more likely it is that you'll have an encounter (or two) with small amounts of feces. However, people with poor diets, high stress levels, and certain medical issues may have more feces in their rectal area even after a bowel movement. If that's the case for you or your partner, you may want to consider having an enema before you engage in anal play.

Shower and wash both your genitals and anal area before sex. Use a mild soap, if possible. If you're brave, you can even insert your finger about an inch or two into your anal canal and gently clean it out. Keep baby wipes handy for easy cleanup during anal play.

Grab your lube. Unlike the vagina, the rectal area isn't naturally lubricated. That's why it's important to have lubricant on hand, even for external play. Use a thick lubricant to protect the rectum's sensitive tissue. Water-based lubricants can dry out quickly, so I recommend using a silicone-based lubricant for anal play, because it's relatively thick and won't dry out. That said, it's also harder to clean up and can damage some sex toys, so use a condom if you're going to pair a silicone-based lubricant with a toy.

Learn how to relax. If you're going to have anal sex, it's important to teach yourself how to relax beforehand. Learning deep-breathing and muscle relaxation techniques can help if you become anxious or feel your body tightening during sex. Even with relaxation techniques, don't go beyond where you are comfortable. It is your body's way of telling you it isn't ready. If you get tense or the sensations become uncomfortable, tell your partner to stop. When you feel relaxed you can start again—slowly.

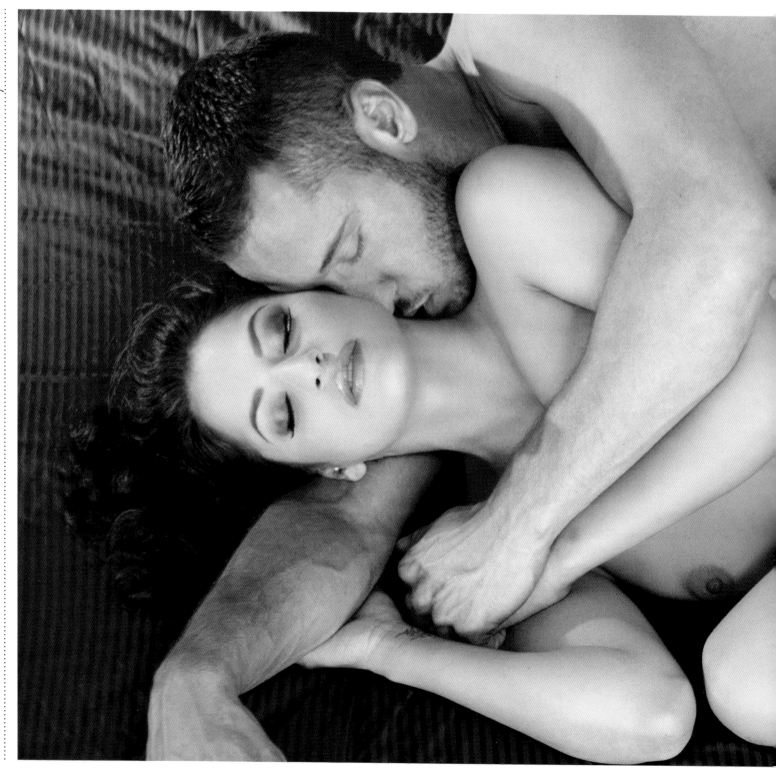

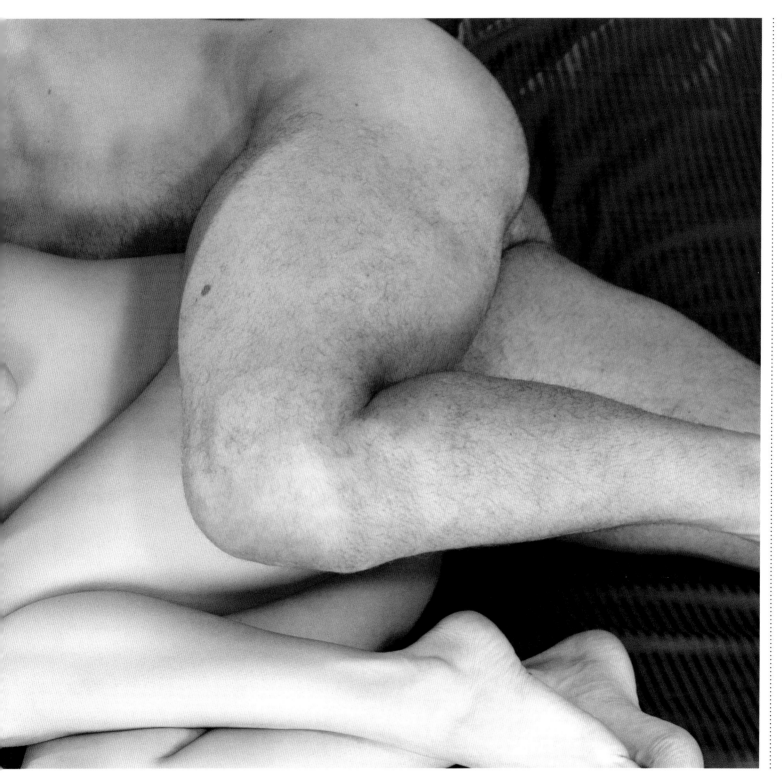

Start by being conscious of your breath. After a few breaths, try a four-second inhale-exhale. Taking long breaths may feel uncomfortable at first, but if you do it regularly when you're anxious, you'll feel your body relax naturally. Being mindful of your muscles is a learning process. It teaches you how your muscles feel when they're tense, and how they feel when they're relaxed. Once you know the difference, you'll be able to tell when your body is responding to your emotions—before a sexual encounter, in a meeting at work, or anywhere else you tend to feel anxious. Starting with your lower body—feet, calves, and thighs—tense one muscle, then relax it. Repeat the process a few times, and be aware of how each muscle feels when it's tensed and relaxed. Slowly work your way up your body—to your buttocks, abdominals, shoulders, neck, and face. By the time you reach your face, your body will be far more relaxed than it was when you started.

Communicate. Great communication before, during, and after anal sex is essential. Take the time to talk to your partner about how you feel about anal sex before you do it. What are your opinions, concerns, and desires? Set verbal boundaries with each other, and choose a "safe" word or signal that you can use if you want to stop. Keep talking during sex, too: be sure to voice both positive and negative feelings. Again, anal sex needs to be approached slowly and with the utmost respect for your body's signals. Whether you are a first-timer or participate in anal play regularly, *always* ask your partner to stop or slow down if things become uncomfortable or if your body isn't relaxed and ready for more.

GOING ALL THE WAY: ANAL PENETRATION

Now that you've become comfortable with anal play and you know what to expect from anal sex, it might be time to progress to penile penetration. Here's how to start: have your partner slowly push his erect penis against your anus while massaging your anal area with his finger at the same time. (Remember: Make sure you have plenty of that silicone-based lubricant on hand.) If he's watching, he'll be able to see your sphincter muscles contract—the anus will tighten and then release, similar to the wink of an eye. When your anus relaxes, he can enter you. Take a deep breath, and, as you exhale, have your partner slowly push his penis into your anus. Meanwhile, either you or your partner should stimulate your clitoris to help keep you aroused. Doing so will allow you to relax and enjoy the anal penetration. (Some women also find that double penetration can be pleasurable. Try it by inserting a finger into one orifice—either your vagina or your anus—and his penis in the other.) After the initial penetration, go slowly, and tell him to move as slowly as you need him to. Don't rush. You're dealing with a very delicate part of your body, so anal sex takes small, gradual steps.

When you first begin experimenting with anal sex, try to use positions in which you're facing each other, or other positions in which you're able to communicate easily with your partner. Each position will be a learning experience. Take your time, and figure out what works best for you.

MISSIONARY

Place a pillow under your hips to elevate your buttocks so that he'll have easier access to your anus. Lie on your back, and have him enter you while he's on top. Then, you can put your legs around him or on his shoulders. You might find that it's easier if you lie on the edge of the bed while he stands or kneels next to it.

Benefits

This position gives you full eye and face contact. Your partner will be able to see your physical reactions for himself, so he'll quickly know whether you're feeling pleasure or discomfort.

Challenges

The missionary position allows for deep penetration, so be careful and go slowly.

Variations and Tips

Place your legs on your partner's chest or over his shoulders. This elevates your anus, which gives him easier access and a great view while it increases your comfort level. You can also place a pillow under your hips for more intense penetration.

SPOONING

You and your partner both lie on your sides, facing the same direction. He inserts his penis into your anus.

Benefits

This is a more comfortable position, and may be easier to relax into, so it's a good choice for your first time. Both you and your partner will enjoy good control over both the angle and the depth of the penetration. The side-by-side spooning position allows for a long, comfortable anal sex session, and leaves his hands free to roam over your body and clitoris.

Challenges

This position does not allow very deep penetration.

Variations and Tips

While lying on your side, try to bring your knees up to your chest and have him curl his legs around yours for an intimate, hug-like position.

WOMAN ON TOP

Face your partner and straddle him. Keeping your arms straight to support your body weight, lower your anus over his penis. You can bend your knees or stretch your legs straight out in front of you.

Benefits

Woman on Top makes it easy for you to communicate with your partner during sex, and it allows him to see your expressions of pleasure or discomfort. Your and your partner's hands are free to caress and stimulate each other's bodies—and that can only make things hotter. Plus, because you're on top, you are in control of the angle and depth of penetration.

Challenges

You're in control in this position—but you also have to do all the work. Finding the best angle for penetration and supporting your body weight with your legs can be tough.

Variations and Tips

Turn your back to him and try a Reverse Cowgirl. Depending on the angle of his penis, this may be more comfortable for you. This variation makes it easier for you to play with your clitoris, which helps keep you aroused. Communication may be a little more difficult in this position because you're facing away from your partner, so you might want to gain a little experience before you try the Reverse Cowgirl.

REAR ENTRY

You are on your hands and knees, on either the bed or the floor, while your partner penetrates you from behind.

Benefits

In this position, the rectum is usually kept straight, which allows easier control over depth and a deeper level of penetration. It's also possible for him to stimulate your G-spot from this position.

Challenges

While you can both move your hips in this position, your partner has more control, so it is important that you trust him to move at the speed and intensity levels that work for you.

Variations and Tips

Try lying on your stomach while your partner penetrates you from behind. It may be a bit more difficult to find the most comfortable angle in this position—plus, it yields deeper penetration—so it's not for beginners.

ANAL PLAY ON HIM

Like women, each man has his own comfort level when it comes to anal play—but most men do enjoy some level of stimulation in or around the anal area. If you want to help him explore anal stimulation, try using your finger to put light pressure on his perineum, and then around or on his anus. Watch his face for cues of pleasure and excitement. Then, using lubricant or saliva, try inserting your finger into his anus up to the first knuckle. You can try this while you're giving him oral sex, or during vaginal penetration. If you're adding anal play to oral sex, venture south slowly. Be sure to start with his perineum, and then move down to his anus. Now you can lick your finger and then slip it inside him. If that goes well, talk to your partner about how he felt, and together you can decide whether to take things further.

Most men who enjoy anal play prefer oral stimulation and a little finger penetration, but some men are open to even more. A vibrator can feel just as good on him as it does on you. Try using a vibrator on the outside of the anus and on and around his testicles: it'll give him pleasure and can help him relax. If your partner wants to experiment even further, you might try pegging, or stimulating the anus with a dildo or strap-on device. Your partner might find it enjoyable because it stimulates the prostate gland. For more information on and instructions for pegging, check out *Bend Over Boyfriend*, an educational video that features heterosexual couples engaging in male anal penetration. It was made and released by Jackie Strano, owner of Good Vibrations, a San Francisco–based sex-positive sex shop. Check out www.fatalemedia.com.

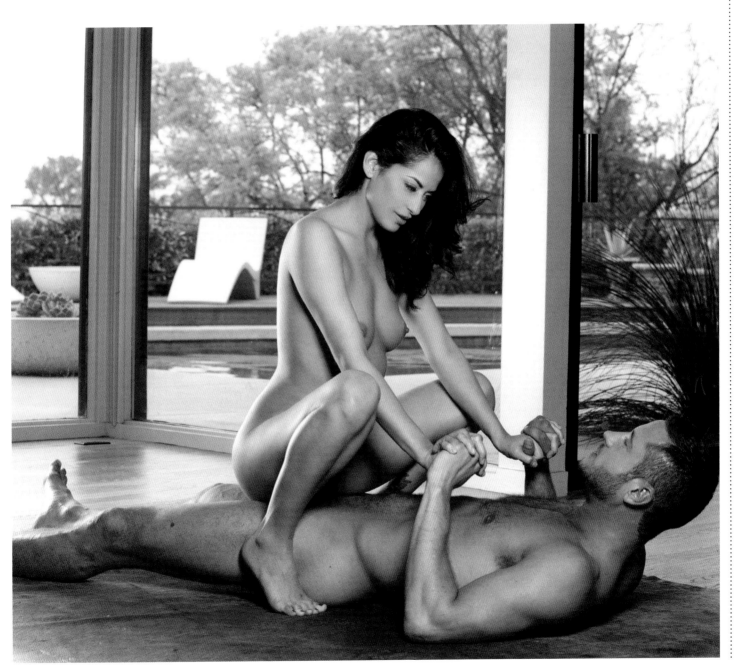

ANAL SEX: ONE WOMAN'S STORY

Each woman comes to her own conclusions about anal sex after experimenting with it. For some women, it can be very pleasurable. Kirsty, thirty-seven, found that anal sex became an important part of her sexuality.

"I was in a relationship at the age of twenty, and had been watching porn, which convinced me that anal sex must be pleasurable. I was young and eager to impress my partner with something new: I thought that if I were into experimentation, my partner would see me as someone who would try anything for him, and would be less likely to leave me. Later, I learned that he was less than impressed with my sexual experimentation: it turned out that I was the one truly getting excited by our sexual adventures. After we had a bad experience while trying anal sex in a hot tub, we were both put off by it, and stopped trying.

"I tried it again later on, and while it was a bit painful, I was convinced that it was supposed to be pleasurable, so I kept trying to make it work. I used a lot of lube and worked on my breathing techniques. Once I taught myself to breathe properly and to relax once the head of his penis was inside me, I noticed that it became less painful and more pleasurable. I was also aroused by how naughty it felt. By my mid-twenties, this became my preferred route to orgasm. I had my system perfected: lube up, align the head of his penis with my anus, concentrate on breathing, and ease him into my ass. I would tell him not to move, and to talk dirty. If he pushed himself into me, it would be painful, but when I was able to control the penetration, it was painless, and I was able to orgasm through anal sex. One of my favorite experiences was when my partner inserted a dildo into my vagina as we had anal sex. As he penetrated me, his scrotum helped to push the dildo further into my vagina.

"Still, I have had a few issues with anal sex. First, I notice that when I introduce it into a relationship, my partner seems to want it all the time. Second, in my twenties, I experienced constipation, bleeding, and the inability to hold in flatulence. When I stopped engaging in anal sex, those issues improved.

"As of now, it has been a few years since I've had anal sex. I'm still interested in it, but am hoping to find a partner with whom I have a deep connection in order to bring the sex to a more connective and intimate place."

SAFETY PRECAUTIONS AND RISKS

In a 2010 study, about half of the women who had tried anal sex reported that it was unpleasant and said they wouldn't want to repeat it. That's fair enough. But that also means that half of the women who tried it were open to trying it a second time, or to experimenting with anal play in other ways. Each woman's body reacts differently to anal sex, so it's important to stick with what's comfortable for you. Because anal tissue isn't as elastic or as moist as the vagina, having anal sex does increase certain health risks, and is more likely to be painful than vaginal sex. Here are some of the most important anal sex safety and risk issues, and how to minimize them:

1. Tears in anal tissue. Because anal tissue is less elastic than vaginal tissue, it's more subject to microtears during penetration. These tiny tears in anal tissue may not produce visible blood or wounds, but they're still dangerous because they can cause tissue damage and transmit diseases. You're thirty times more likely to contract HIV during unprotected anal sex than you are during unprotected vaginal sex. To reduce your risks, have your partner wear a condom, always use lubricant, and talk to your partner about getting tested.

2. Other physical damage. Repetitive physical damage to the rectal area can result in physical issues such as a prolapsed anus or hemorrhoids. It's not as much fun as it sounds, so, to prevent an anal prolapse, do Kegel exercises. They'll help strengthen the muscles and tissue around the anal area. (See page 48 for a crash course in Kegels.)

3. Spread of bacteria. While erotic and pornographic films show couples having oral sex right after anal sex, the simple fact is, anal followed by oral is unsafe. Your rectum contains bacteria that can cause infections in your mouth or vaginal area. If you want to resume vaginal sex or have oral sex after you engage in anal, your partner must wash himself thoroughly first.

4. Hygiene issues. Poor hygiene, like dirty hands, fingers, or anal area, can result in infections and are notorious for spreading bacteria. Long fingernails can cause anal lacerations and infections. To avoid cuts, prior to anal play, trim your fingernails so that they're short and smooth.

In short, anal sex can be safe, enjoyable, and a great way to connect with your partner. It also isn't for everyone and it may not be for you. If so, that's okay! Don't feel like you aren't up to speed if anal sex (or any other sexual act for that matter) is something you don't enjoy and don't want to do. Don't do anal play out of peer or partner pressure. Your body is yours to own for your own pleasure. It's vital that you educate yourself about the risks inherent in anal intercourse or play. Forget about what you see in adult films, as it isn't always accurate: this kind of sex can't be spontaneous or rough, since that approach can be both painful and risky. Remember, there's no such thing as "should" or "shouldn't": use your own judgment when it comes to deciding how much anal play is good for you, your body, and your relationship.

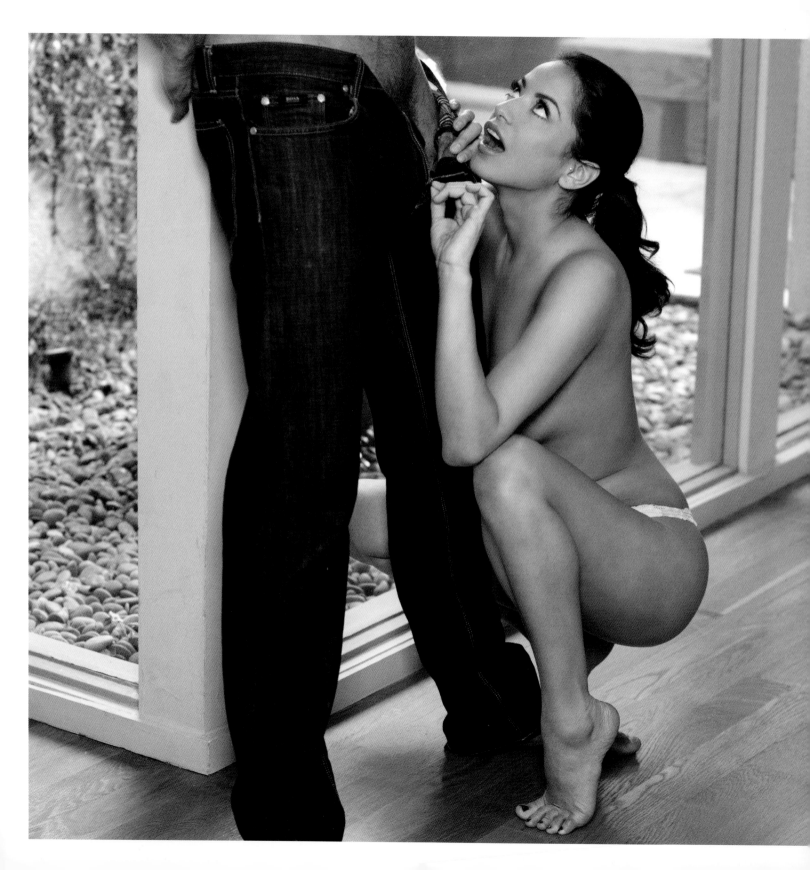

09

Oral Sex: Be Great at Giving It— and Getting It

Whether you're going down on him or he's going down on you, oral sex is much more than a one-sided favor. Giving oral sex can be just as gratifying as getting it, once you know how, and it's an experience that can be incredibly erotic and intimate for both of you. Plus, it's super-versatile: it's enjoyable on its own, but it can also be an "appetizer" to be savored before vaginal sex; it feels good for both of you; and, of course, it's a great way to reach climax.

It's completely okay to feel anxious about performing oral sex—especially if you're doing it with a new partner for the first time. Maybe you don't consider yourself an expert, and you're having doubts about your skills. But that doesn't have to shake your confidence. With a very few exceptions that might result in pain or injury—such as biting the penis too hard, using too firm a grip on it, or bending it—the average man will love just about anything you do with his member. And he'll be especially turned on when you put it in your mouth. Mouth stimulation is really pleasurable, since your mouth comes equipped with a very special tool: your tongue. And it's also an exciting visual experience for him. He gets to watch his penis slide into your sexy mouth, and he can see your facial expressions as you go down on him. What's not to like? That said, in the same way that every woman prefers a different style and type of oral sex, each man will have his own preferences too. That's why communication is the most important sexual skill. You'll learn what he likes by asking him and by paying attention to his verbal and physical cues, such as moans or curling toes.

FOUR STEPS TO A MIND-BLOWING BLOW JOB

Giving oral sex can be empowering for you, too. Just like the Woman on Top sexual position, you're in complete control of the rhythm, duration, speed, and intensity of oral sex, and his penis is, quite literally, completely in your hands (and your mouth, of course). You have the power to bring your partner to orgasm, to delay his orgasm, or to prevent it entirely.

There are four key components when it comes to giving a great blow job, and it's especially handy to remember them if you're new to the game. Just like driving a car, you might feel as if you're overthinking what you're doing at first, but don't worry. It'll soon feel much more natural.

STEP 1: THE TEASE

The tease is all about how you want to initiate the encounter. Some women are perfectly comfortable with grabbing his penis and getting to work ASAP, but you may not be. That's fine. Besides, teasing gets him aroused and puts you both in the mood. (You may even enjoy the tease more than the act itself!) So enjoy building the anticipation. Occasionally, it can be exciting when you grab him, unzip him, and get down to business, but try not to take the bull by the horns (or horn) too often. If you don't build anticipation into the experience, the act will become predictable—and, over time, that'll get boring for both him and you.

Start with your hands. As you're kissing your partner, use your hands to caress and rub the area around his groin, and work your way up to fondling his penis. You'll know whether he's enjoying it from the sounds, motions, and gestures he makes, and from his direct verbal responses. Every man is different: some men may respond by moaning, others by breathing heavily, and others might tell you exactly what they like.

(If he doesn't tell you directly, feel free to ask him. Hearing him tell you that he likes what you're doing can make any kind of sex even hotter.) You might start by lightly caressing his penis before you grasp it more firmly through his underwear or pants. At this point, it's likely that his penis will be mostly or completely erect. That can be a huge turn-on for you. After all, it's empowering to know that your attractiveness and your skilled touch are responsible for his arousal.

Now move your mouth south. Move the action along at the speed that feels comfortable for you—but you might want to go slowly if this is a first encounter, or if you simply want to draw out the seduction to make it last as long as possible. Continue kissing your partner, then let your lips and tongue slowly work their way down his body, from his neck, chest, and nipples to his stomach. Finally, when you're near his penis, use your mouth and hands to caress and lick the skin around and near the penis and testicles—but avoid the penis itself. Try running your fingers and fingernails lightly over his sensitive areas as you move closer and closer to his genitals.

STEP 2: START THE ACTION

Now you're between his legs, and he's aroused and ready for action. What next? Well, there's really no "wrong" way to start. Remember that your mouth isn't the limit: you can use your hands, fingers, mouth, face, lips, and tongue to get the penis's vast amount of nerve endings all hot and bothered. Here are a few suggestions to get going:

Go from hand to mouth. Begin by taking his penis in one or both hands and, using a light grasp, move your hand up and down on his shaft as if you were giving him a hand job. Then take the head of the penis in your mouth and, using a circular motion, slowly massage it with your tongue. Remember that the head of the penis is the most sensitive part of his genitals—particularly the frenulum, which is the underside of the head—so be gentle. Don't stop moving your hands while his penis is in your mouth. Use one or both hands as an extension of your mouth: run them straight up and down the shaft, or twist your hands lightly to switch up the sensation. If you're using one hand, try using the other to rub his chest, massage his thigh, or lightly cup and caress his testicles. Or, put that free hand to good use by stroking your own body or masturbating: it's exciting for you and really visually arousing for him.

Tease, tease, suck. Another way to start is by running your tongue vertically along the shaft of his penis, then turning your head to apply your lips to his shaft in a wide kissing motion. After teasing the shaft a little, move your mouth to the head of his penis and lick, kiss, and suck the head before taking the entire penis in your mouth.

STEP 3: KEEP IT UP

This step is the meat of the blow job. (Pun very much intended.) It's where the main action happens, and it's when you bring him to climax or not, depending on how you want to progress with the sex act. For example, maybe you're planning to move on to vaginal sex, and the blow job is a warm-up act. These are the moments when you have complete control, so enjoy them, and get creative. Your blow job doesn't have to be all about the tongue: your mouth is an immensely complicated, intricate, and multifaceted part of your body, and it can create incredibly varied sensations for your partner. Rub or lightly suck his member with your lips. Gently nibble the head of the penis with your teeth. Hold the penis against the side of your cheek to give him a different sensation of suction. To increase the intensity of the moment that you take his penis into your mouth, try making, and holding, eye contact with him. Men tend to be visual in nature, so part of the sexual experience for him is what he *sees* you do.

Go all the way. While the most sensitive part of the penis is its head, it can be really visually arousing for your partner to watch you take nearly the full length of his penis in your mouth. Place your mouth around the head of his penis and slowly proceed down the shaft, making eye contact with him all the time. There's no need to be too ambitious in terms of depth (we'll discuss "deep-throating" later on in this chapter).

You set the pace. The rhythm and speed of the blow job are up to you, and you can adjust both depending on your partner's responses. Generally, it's a good idea to start with a slow, rhythmic motion and increase the speed over the duration of the encounter.

One hand or two? As you move your mouth up and down over the head and shaft of his penis, you can use one or both hands to create extra sensation for your partner. Move them up and down the shaft in a straight, vertical motion, or twist your hands slightly as they slide up and down. Make sure both your hands and mouth are well lubricated to prevent painful friction.

Getting tired? If you're going for orgasm with your blow job, rather than using it as a warm-up to intercourse, your hands, mouth, jaw, and neck may get tired after a while. Here's how to give yourself a break without stopping the action. If your hands get tired, place them on his thighs or chest, and use only your mouth. This gives your hands a rest, but he won't notice because he'll be too excited by the clear view of his penis in your mouth. Or gently rub his penis around your mouth, then remove it and move it down your chest to your breasts. You can squeeze your breasts together to masturbate his penis, or you can tantalize him by rubbing it against your breasts. If your mouth or jaw gets tired, throw your head back and use only your hands while continuing to look him in the eyes. This can feel really empowering, because you have complete control over him and, by locking eyes with him, you're letting him know it. Use your hands for as long as you need to, and feel free to mix things up by alternating hands, massaging his testicles, spitting on his penis for lubrication, and occasionally focusing on the head only. If your neck gets tired during the blow job, use the technique for a tired mouth, or change your position. You can give oral sex in a reverse position on top, while kneeling before him, lying horizontally next to him, or even standing over him.

"If giving oral sex is hard because his penis is too big, or because you're getting tired, it's okay to take a break. Remember that you are in control. Push the penis away, pull your head back, take a deep breath, and exhale while making eye contact with him. Use what you think is a disadvantage to your advantage to make it hot and sexy."

—Lia, Vivid contract girl and *Penthouse* model

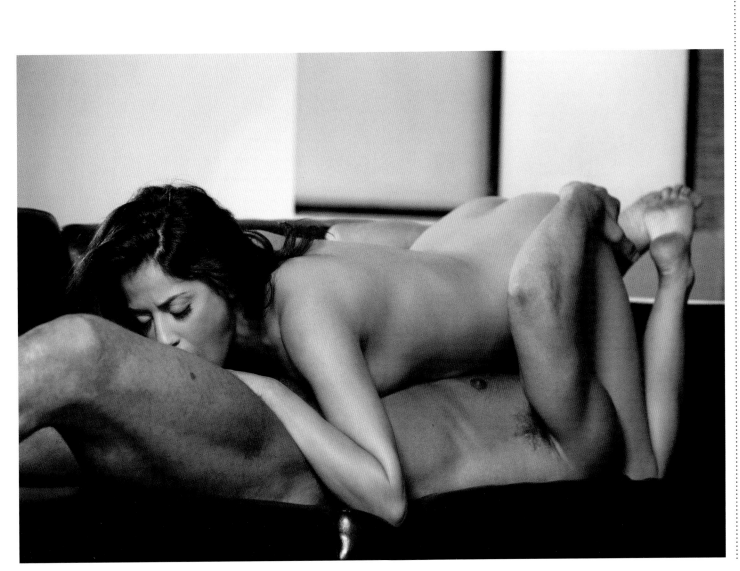

"I really don't have any magic blow job tricks. I have a very small gag reflex—I know: I'm a porn star and I can't deep-throat. Weird, right?— so I use my hands a lot and I use a lot of spit. And I treat the penis like my own lollipop— and I just have fun."
—Joanna Angel, adult actress/director, *Burning Angel*

STEP 4: GO PAST THE SHAFT

Blow jobs don't have to focus on the head and shaft of his penis only. When you're going down on him, pay attention to the surrounding areas. After all, his entire package is fair game here. Explore the areas around the penis, and note his reactions. If you hear moans, see toes curling, or feel him breathe rapidly, keep going! Try tantalizing his …

Testicles and perineum. The testicles and the area around them are highly sensitive for most men. Start by licking, kissing, and caressing the area around the testicles, and then run your fingers over his testicles and the perineum. (The perineum is the area between his balls and his anus, and it's highly sensitive to touch.) Licking the testicles and perineum is usually very pleasurable, and he'll probably love it if you suck on his testicles lightly. Try taking each testicle in your mouth, and suck and massage it with your tongue. Lick his perineum while you continue to use your hands to stroke the shaft or testicles. Alternate soft, wet licks with targeted pressure, and press your tongue firmly against the perineum.

Anal area. If you're feeling adventurous, try moving your tongue or fingers south to his anal area. (Some men love anal play, while others don't. You can ask your partner directly whether he likes to be licked or touched there, or you can move slowly toward the area and see how he responds. Be mindful of his verbal and physical responses.) Start by lightly running your fingers around the perimeter of his anus. Move your tongue from the perineum to the anus and circle it, using only very light pressure. Remember, you can stop and continue the oral sex any time by moving back to his testicles or penis. Anal play can be enjoyed safely by using a latex glove and dental dam. Always wash your hands with antibacterial soap and hot water before and after anal play. For a full rundown on how to enjoy back-door play, see chapter 8.

"What are the keys to a great blow job? Confidence, feeling hot, saliva, and eye contact. In that order." —Lia, Vivid contract girl and *Penthouse* model

DEEP-THROATING

First of all, what is it? Deep-throating is the act of taking the penis past your epiglottis—the flap of cartilage that's visible at the back of your mouth—and further into your throat. It's definitely a skill that requires practice, and you really have to want to do it. Most women experience an issue with the gag reflex the first few times they try it—but, with practice, you can train yourself to suppress it. Why does it feel good for your partner? Because when the head of the penis is pressed toward the back of your throat, the resulting sensation of tightness is really pleasurable. As with all fellatio, the woman is completely in charge when it comes to deep-throating. You can work it into oral sex for only a moment, or you can prolong it and turn it into an act in itself. It depends, first and foremost, on what you're comfortable with.

Several positions work well for deep-throating. Just as a sword swallower "swallows" a sword by keeping his throat straight, deep-throating works well when your throat is straight and your neck isn't curved. Try this position: lie with your head hanging off of the edge of the bed, and have your partner enter your mouth while he's standing. Go slowly, and be sure to decide beforehand on a safety signal you can give your partner if it gets too intense, such as a hand gesture or two taps to the side of the leg. Like any other sex act, experiment and find out what works best for you. And remember, you don't have to be able to deep-throat to give a great blow job.

WHAT TO DO WHEN HE COMES

It's a good idea to think in advance about what you're comfortable with when it comes to your partner's orgasm. While it's best to talk to your partner about what turns you on and what your limitations are, that's easier said than done, particularly when you're in the heat of the moment, if or the relationship is new. You know all about male ejaculation from reading chapter 6, so you know that your partner will typically reach orgasm within five to ten minutes of stimulation. So, what do you when he comes? There are different ways to engage with his orgasm that can be pleasurable for both of you. You might choose to swallow his semen, but if you're not comfortable with that, it's okay to spit it out. You can also take his penis out of your mouth as he's about to come and bring him to climax in your hands, on your body, inside your vagina, or on his own body. Whatever you decide, it's completely up to you.

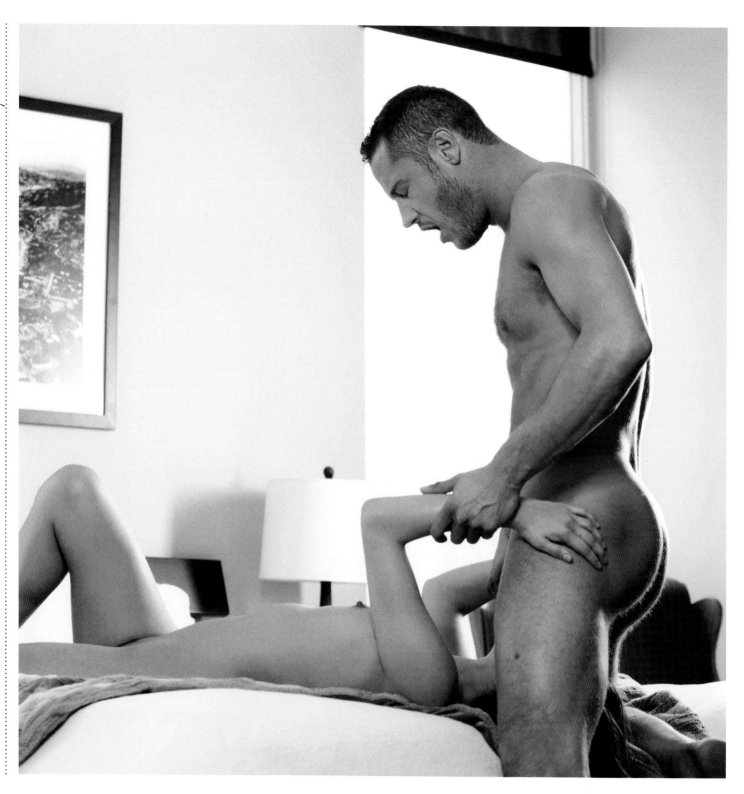

ORAL SEX: A FULL-BODY EXPERIENCE

When you're giving oral sex, it's easy to focus so much on his penis that you forget about the rest of his body. It's tempting to be penis-centric—but that can make sex one-dimensional and, more often than not, boring. Being mindful of his entire body can be pleasurable for both of you. Stoke his excitement by caressing his chest, hands, legs, and face while your mouth is attending to his penis. Take a quick break from oral sex to make eye contact with him and kiss him. Use one of your hands to stroke his shaft while holding his hand with the other. Or, as you're going down on him, let your hand glide down his chest and let it rest over his heart. Details like these move oral sex beyond a mechanical act to an erotic, emotionally connected exchange that's enjoyable for both parties. Great sex is always a full-body, *shared* experience—even when you're performing oral sex on him.

PAY ATTENTION TO HIS PHYSICAL AND VERBAL CUES

How do you know whether he likes what you're doing? While you're going down on him, pay attention to his physical and verbal cues. You'll know he's into it if you notice physical signs, such as heavy breathing, perspiration, muscle twitching or spasms, pointing or flexing his feet or toes, feeling him grip your body firmly with his hands, seeing his pelvis lift, or changes in his facial expressions and eye contact. Or he might respond verbally, either through words or groans. If he groans in response to your movements, you'll know you're doing a great job. He might also tell you explicitly that he likes what you're doing. If he doesn't, that's okay. Take it upon yourself to ask. Asking him directly is a great idea for two reasons: you'll find out which moves work best for him, and you'll both be turned on by hearing him express his pleasure out loud. So don't be afraid to speak up. Tell him what you like about giving him oral sex, and what the hottest part of the experience is for you. He'll love it—seeing you excited will be exciting to him.

CUNNILINGUS: FEEL CONFIDENT WHEN HE'S GOING DOWN ON YOU

Most women need clitoral stimulation to achieve orgasm. A lot of intercourse positions and the way your body "fits" with your partner's can make direct clitoral stimulation a challenge—but oral sex gives your partner direct access to your clitoris, making orgasm more likely. So, if you don't come easily during intercourse, oral sex can be a great way to get yours. But what if you don't feel as good about getting as you do about giving? It's funny: in the same way that there are hundreds of books and online tutorials telling women how to perform great fellatio, there's also a huge amount of information aimed at men on how to give great cunnilingus. But despite the vast amount of information available on *giving* oral sex, there's precious little out there for women on how to feel confident *receiving* oral sex. And it doesn't help that lots of women feel anxious about it—especially when it comes to how their vaginas look, smell, taste, and feel to their partners. (If you need a confidence boost when it comes to your lady parts, reread chapter 3: Boosting Your Sexual Self-Esteem.) Don't worry: the fact is, all vaginas are unique, and there's no such thing as a "negative" vaginal attribute unless it's something that compromises your health. Here are some great ways to participate actively when he goes down on you.

HOW TO GET WHAT YOU WANT FROM ORAL SEX

While it may seem like he's in the driver's seat during cunnilingus—and some women love oral sex for precisely that reason—there are a number of things you can do to get the most out of the experience.

Guide him with your hands. Point to show him where you want him to go, or gently move his head in the right direction.

Provide easy access. To help him reach your vagina, place a pillow under your hips. That'll raise your entire pubic area, which gives him easier access to you.

Get on top. Straddle him and hover over his mouth as he goes down on you. In this position, you'll be able to move freely and easily and control pressure and speed.

Know yourself. Being in tune with your own body will help you guide him when he's giving you oral sex—and the best way to find out what you like is to masturbate. There's lots more on masturbation in chapter 3, but here are some tips for finding out what feels good to you.

• *Consider shaving or waxing.* Some women find that shaving or waxing their pubic hair, especially around the labia, can increase sensation and can allow them to see their vaginal parts more easily.

• *Get wet.* Take a long, hot bath and see how the water feels as it streams over your vulva. Use that as a benchmark for what feels good.

• *Use a mirror.* Grab a mirror, preferably one that stands up by itself, and check out your vagina. Look at yourself as you touch and explore. Move from the outer labia, inner labia, clitoral area, and vaginal opening toward your anus.

STAYING LUBRICATED DURING ORAL SEX

A woman's natural vaginal lubrication can fluctuate throughout her life, depending on things like oral contraceptives, hormonal changes, and arousal levels. Even if you're perfectly healthy, you might find that staying lubricated is an issue from time to time, and that can make oral sex less enjoyable. But solutions are at hand. Encourage your partner to moisten his fingers and mouth with saliva before and during oral sex. During sex, if you feel you still need lubrication, lick your own fingers and moisten the outside of your vagina with your saliva—or, if you're feeling more aggressive, place two fingers in your partner's mouth, then insert those fingers into your vagina.

You can also buy lubricants that are made specifically for oral sex, including flavored ones. It's fine to use these, too: just be sure to wash your genitals after sex, because some of them contain sugars that can lead to yeast infections.

TELL HIM—AND SHOW HIM— WHAT YOU LIKE

In the same way that a woman might feel insecure about performing fellatio on her partner, men also worry about their skills when it comes to cunnilingus. Naturally, every woman has her own preferences, turn-ons and turn-offs, and ways to reach orgasm. So, the best way to enjoy yourself when he's giving you oral sex is to tell and show him what works for you. You'll figure out what you like and what you don't through masturbation: it's important to know and love your body both for yourself and so you can coach your partner on what you want during oral sex. Using verbal and visual cues will tell him that he's on the right track when he's going down on you.

Verbal cues are things you say or sounds you make to show him that he's pleasuring you. The sighs, moans, and deep breathing that come naturally to you when you're aroused tell him that you like what he's doing. Don't feel like you have to fake it, though. If you feel inclined to make noise, go with it and let your instincts guide you. You can also let your partner know what you want by telling him directly. For instance, you could simply tell him you like it when he licks your clitoris. Or you can give him instructions— say that you want him to use his fingers and his tongue at the same time. Giving him direct instructions can really heighten the experience for both of you because it can feel empowering for you and arousing for him. (Plus, you're sure to get exactly what you want!) So speak up. If you want him to do something different, just tell him.

Physical cues are also a great way to subtly coach your partner. Using your body to show him that he's pleasing you will help him feel more confident, and will encourage him to keep doing what he's doing. If you feel the urge to move your body as he's going down on you, don't hold back. Do it uninhibitedly. After all, it's normal for a woman to move her hips and writhe around when she's aroused. And, if you want to encourage your lover to go further south, let your own hands and fingers travel there first. This shows him exactly where you want to be touched. You can also put gentle pressure on his shoulders or head to let him know that you want him between your legs. As he moves lower, massage his shoulders and head as positive reinforcement. When his mouth is between your legs, it's time to lie back, relax, and enjoy being on the receiving end of oral sex—but be sure to interact with him throughout. If you want him to focus more on the clitoris, for example, place your hands around it, point to it, or stimulate it yourself. If you want your partner to move below your vagina to your perineum or anal area, lift your hips and pelvis up to guide him in the right direction.

GREAT POSITIONS FOR CUNNILINGUS

You're well versed in sex positions that involve penile penetration—you've read chapter 7!—but did you know that there are also a number of different positions when it comes to cunnilingus? Here are a few of the best:

Woman on her back, partner lying or kneeling between her legs. Simply lie on your back, spread your legs, and let him get to work. This position gives him easy access to your vaginal area—plus, it's relaxing and comfortable for you. You can put a pillow under your hips for your comfort and to give him greater access to your lady parts.

Woman on top—or "face-sitting." In this position, you can face forward or backward, whichever works for you, and you can avoid putting all of your weight on him by kneeling over him and lowering your vulva over his face. This does require thigh strength, so if you haven't been doing your lunges lately, try bending over and resting your straight arms on his body to help support yourself. This position is comfortable for him, and it gives you plenty of control in terms of depth of oral penetration and pelvic movement. It also frees up your hands so that you can pleasure yourself or masturbate your partner if you're facing backward.

69. Reverse Cowgirl is also a great way to ease into a 69 position, which allows simultaneous oral stimulation. If your partner is much larger or heavier than you are, 69 might be easier if you're on top—plus, you'll be able to move around more freely. Having him on top is also an option, but do encourage your partner to kneel over you to reduce the pressure of his weight and his penis. Try 69 while you're lying side by side for another alternative. In this position, both partners can lie flat, and it's easy to rest your head on a pillow or your partner's leg.

STAY SAFE AND HEALTHY DURING ORAL SEX

Unprotected oral sex is a safer type of sexual interaction than unprotected vaginal or anal sex, but it's still important to know the risks. HIV can be transmitted through cuts in the genitals or mouth, as well as through ejaculation. Both type 1 and type 2 herpes can be passed on via oral sex, as can HPV, the virus that causes genital warts and cervical cancers. In fact, some new studies support the theory that HPV (which is passed from skin to skin and not through bodily fluids) that's contracted through oral sex may even be responsible for some types of throat cancers. Gonorrhea and chlamydia can be transmitted via oral sex, and they can manifest in the throat, where treatment can be difficult, and syphilis can also be contracted through oral sex. So be sure to protect yourself, especially if you're having oral sex with a new partner. Use a condom or dental dam to minimize risks. (See chapter 1 for more on STIs and how to reduce your risk of contracting them.)

Whether you're on the giving or receiving end, oral sex can be an arousing, satisfying, intimate experience for you both. Now that you're up on going down, read on to find out how sex toys for you (and him!), erotica, and even porn can turn up the heat in your sex life.

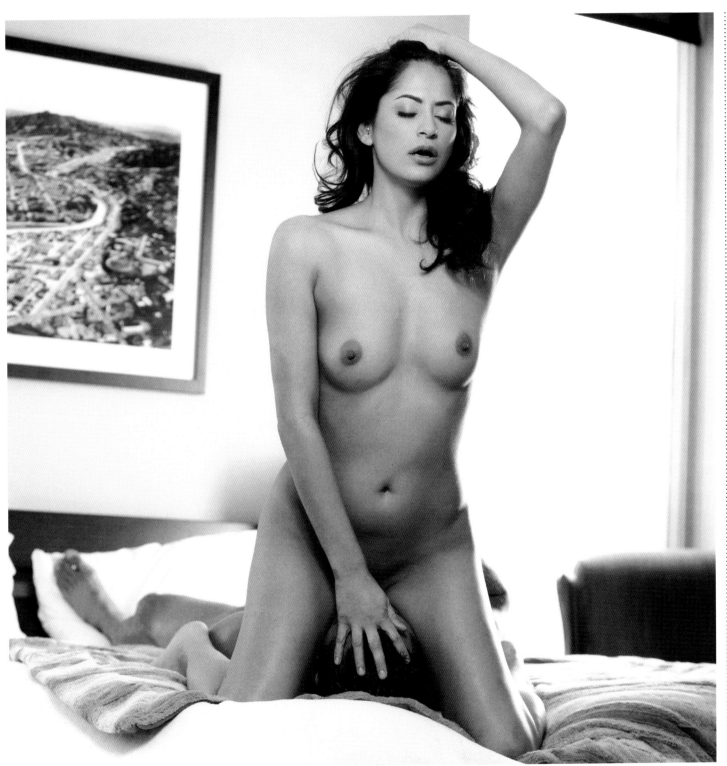

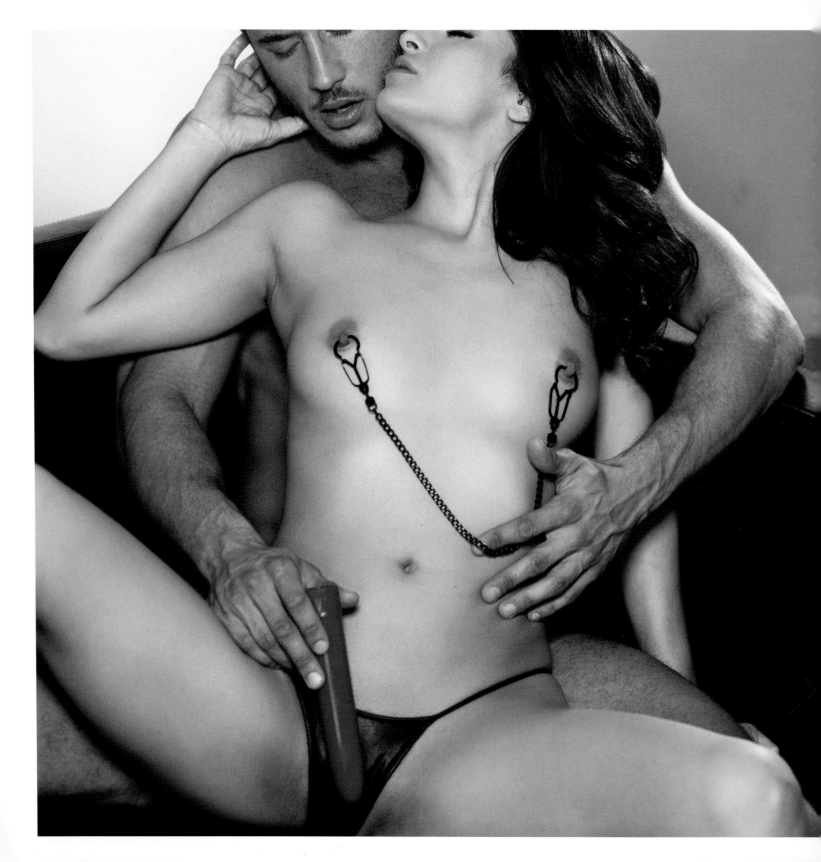

10 ☿ *Sex Toys: Tools of the Trade*

Sex toys, erotica, adult videos, and porn can all be great ways to add new dimensions to your sex life. But getting your hands on them can be a challenge. For instance, when I was a teenager, my hometown had a single, windowless adult-themed store. As I drove by, I used to wonder at the devious or mysterious things that might be going on in there. No way would I have ever gone inside! More recently, I was approached by a family friend in her sixties who asked me nervously where she could buy her first erotic video. She wanted to spice up her love life with her husband of over thirty years. She went on to tell me that she had been too embarrassed to buy the lubricant that her physician recommended, and the water-based product she had on hand was sticky and uncomfortable to use. She felt lost and defeated—and I was glad she had turned to me for help.

These situations are really common. How do you find sex toys, erotic material like porn or adult videos, or simply products to help make sex more comfortable? And how do you know what to buy? This chapter has the answers. It'll give you the lowdown on sex toys for you and your partner—and it'll tell you how to use them. Plus, you'll find out why watching porn can be great for your sex life, whether you're solo or part of a couple and, most important, where to find the good stuff. Let's start with sex toys.

WHY SHOULD I TRY SEX TOYS?

Sex toys are handheld devices that are made to give you sexual pleasure. Whether you're single or in a relationship, there are lots of reasons to experiment with sex toys. First, they can offer clitoral stimulation. Most women can orgasm more easily through clitoral stimulation—but some intercourse positions don't allow easy access to the clitoris. Using a sex toy during intercourse can help you reach orgasm. Many toys can help you reach orgasm faster—and, sometimes, more intensely. And that means more pleasure, whether you're alone or à deux. For instance, while he's penetrating you, try using a vibrator on your clitoris to achieve a blended orgasm.

Sex toys are also great tools for increasing your body awareness, which can help you be a better lover and get more out of sex. Experimenting with sex toys when you're by yourself lets you figure out what you like, and how you like to be stimulated without the pressure of pleasing a partner or awkwardly fumbling around until you master the technique. It's a no-pressure way to learn about your body or just to experience sexual pleasure. Adding toys to your sexual repertoire means you'll be able to maximize the sexual experiences you can have when you're on your own. You don't necessarily need a partner to enjoy sexual pleasure. Sex toys can be great if you're between sexual partners or your current partner can't have sex for whatever reason.

However, don't forgo buying and experimenting with sex toys as a couple if your partner is willing. Sex toys can add a dimension of kink to your sex play, which is a real turn-on. They're also practical. Sex toys can do the work that hands, lips, and other body parts may be too tired or unable to do.

There are lots of different types of sex toys on the market, and each type is unique in terms of function and benefits. Some offer clitoral stimulation, while others offer penetration or vibration—or a combination of all three. Here's a breakdown of the basic types of toys.

VIBRATORS

A vibrator is a sex toy that pulses rapidly, causing pleasurable sensations for the body, skin, and genitals. Vibrators are usually powered by electricity or batteries. Electric vibrators, such as the Hitachi Magic Wand, tend to be larger and more powerful, and can often be used for full-body massage as well as sexual pleasure. Battery-powered vibrators can be as small as 1 inch (2.5 centimeters) in length, or as long as 12 inches (30 centimeters). The smaller versions, also know as bullets, are small, pocket-size vibrating toys that are best for clitoral stimulation, while larger, vibrating wands, such as the Rabbit, can also be inserted into the vagina. G-spot stimulators are vibrators that are curved so that they stimulate your G-spot with pressure and vibration once they're inserted.

HOW TO USE IT

Super-versatile vibrators can be used in lots of ways. Most of the time, they're used for clitoral stimulation, either solo or during intercourse. But there's no need to focus exclusively on the clitoris: feel free to move the vibrator around your vulva and the surrounding area. Turn the vibrator on and experiment with different motions; notice how it feels on different areas of your genitals and see which pressure levels feel good for you. If it's your first time, try placing a piece of fabric, such as a towel, between your vulva and the toy to reduce the intensity of the vibration.

You can also use your vibrator on your partner's body, especially on his testicles and perineum, and on his anal area. In fact, anal vibration for both partners can be pleasurable. *Just be sure to use a toy with a tapered end*, which prevents it from getting lost inside the rectum. If you're sharing a vibrator, cover it with a condom before using it, and be sure to wash it after each use. Speaking of water, a word to the wise: some vibrators are waterproof, and some aren't, so make sure that your vibrator is made for water exposure before you take it with you into the shower.

BEST PICKS

The Hitachi Magic Wand. Nicknamed the "Cadillac of vibrators," this toy was created to be a handheld massage tool, but became popular as a fabulous sex toy in the 1970s. (Feel free to use it for both!) It also comes with attachments, which give you more options for variation and experimentation.

The Rabbit. The Rabbit is a toy that has a shaft for insertion and a clitoral stimulator that vibrates. It's great for simultaneous internal and external stimulation.

PENIS VS. DILDO?

You may have heard that some men feel
threatened by dildos, especially if they're
larger than the average erect penis. But
the fact is, most men aren't intimated
by sex toys. If your partner doesn't seem
terribly interested when you bring your
battery-powered toy into the bedroom, try
softening the introduction a little. Tell your
partner that, while you enjoy pleasuring
yourself with your sex toy, sex with him is a
different experience that can't be replicated
by anything mechanical. Be open with him:
tell your partner what you like about your toy,
and show him how to use it on you—often
men find using a dildo on their partner quite
exciting. He'll feel more comfortable with
it in no time.

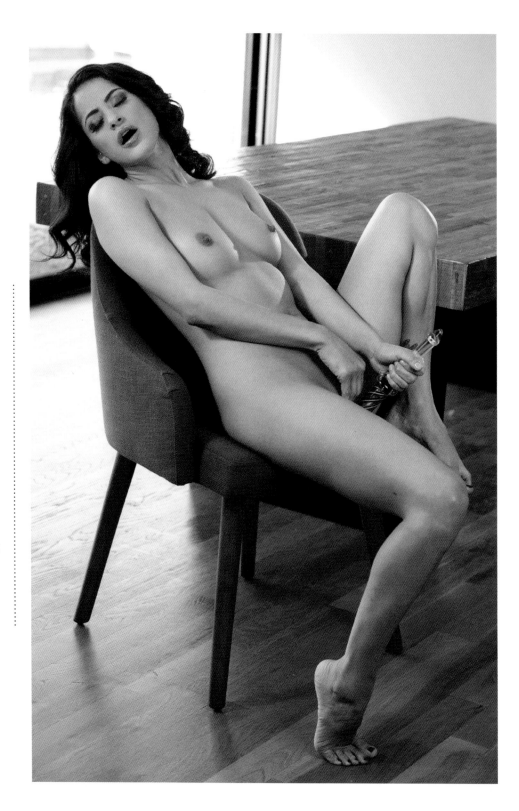

DILDOS

Dildos are phallic (penis-shaped) sex toys that are meant to be inserted into the vagina. There are literally thousands of types of dildos on the market. While some are "realistic" and look like penises, others are smooth and shaped more like a rounded cylinder than an actual penis. They can be made from just about anything—from plastic to silicone to glass. In fact, glass dildos have become increasingly popular, and are sometimes even made from hand-blown glass. These types of dildos are great for easy cleaning, and for anyone who's allergic to latex. Rubber dildos are less expensive, but need to be replaced more often, while glass and metal dildos are more expensive but can last for years.

Dildos come in a range of sizes, and, if you're a first-timer, it's best to start small until you're sure of the size that's right for you. Bigger really isn't always better. A dildo that's too large can be uncomfortable, and that's no fun. Be especially mindful of your dildo's diameter: if you buy a dildo that's too long, you can always insert it only to the point at which it feels good, but if you buy one that's too wide or thick, there isn't much you can do. For G-spot or prostate stimulation, try a curved dildo. Or, for something a bit different, try a dildo with a suction-cup base, which can be mounted on flat surfaces like walls, stable tables, headboards, or shower doors. Suction-cup dildos are great because they allow for hands-free stimulation and penetration, and being hands-free lets you use your hands to massage yourself or to stimulate your clitoris. Here's how to use them: place the dildo on a flat, stable surface, then mount it in the Woman on Top position, just as you'd mount a partner. Or stick it to a wall and use it for rear entry or to practice your oral sex skills. In the shower or bath, stick it to the wall or the floor and indulge in some good clean fun— just be careful not to slip, and be sure to support yourself on a stable wall or hand bar. To get the kinky effect of a threesome, bring your partner into the action.

HOW TO USE IT

Dildos are stationary, and require you to do the work, so to speak. Be sure to have lubricant on hand in case you need it, because you might not be as moist as you would be after foreplay with a partner. If you are using a silicone dildo, use a water-based lubricant only: silicone-based lubricant on a silicone toy will destroy the toy and may make it less safe to use. Start by rubbing the head of the dildo against the outside of your vulva, and be aware of its texture and the sensations that result. Next, insert the toy an inch or two into your vagina. Experiment by twisting it and inserting it at different speeds and at different angles. Gradually, work your way up to inserting the dildo into your vagina at a depth that you're comfortable with. If you feel any pain or discomfort, slow down or stop. When you're using your dildo with your partner, show him how you like to use it when you're alone. Give him the toy, and have him do what you've just shown him. If you're feeling more adventurous, dildos can also be used in a harness as a strap-on.

If you want to try anal play with your dildo, make sure you buy a suitable one. All dildos are good for vaginal penetration, but only some are approved for anal penetration. Dildos meant for anal penetration typically have a flared bottom to prevent the toy from getting lodged in the rectum.

BEST PICKS

Charm Silicone Dildo. Available in 5- or 7-inch (12.7 or 17.8 centimeter) lengths, this silicone toy is recommended as a great starter toy by Good Vibrations sex shop in San Francisco. Because it has a flared end, you can use it either vaginally or anally. Plus, it's harness-compatible if you're interested in using it as a strap-on.

ANAL TOYS

Anal toys are sex toys that are made specifically for use in that sensitive rectal area, and many of them are flared at the end for safety. Anal plugs are smooth, cone-shaped objects that are flared at one end, and they're meant to remain stationary in the rectum. They deliver a pleasurable sense of "fullness" or penetration in the anal area, and, once inserted, they can be left alone. There's no need to move them in and out as you would a dildo. Anal plugs come in many sizes. If you're new to them, get the smallest one possible (which will probably be slightly larger than a finger). Be sure to use lubricant when you insert it (but remember: if the anal plug is silicone, don't use silicone lubricant with it). Anal beads are strings of beads that are inserted into the anal area. They can be left in during intercourse, or slowly pulled out. Proceed with caution, though. Plastic anal beads may have sharp seams. You might want to try anal beads made of silicone instead, because they'll be smoother. *Always* hold on to the end of the string of beads, and don't let them go all the way into your anus. Anal dildos and vibrators are made specifically for anal use. They're usually very smooth and have a flared end. When you're using them on your partner or yourself, always go slowly and use plenty of lubricant.

HOW TO USE THEM

As you would with any sex toy, apply a generous amount of lubricant and slowly insert the toy into your or your partner's anus. Don't forget to communicate: if you're using anal toys on someone else, check in with him from time to time to make sure he's not uncomfortable or experiencing pain.

BEST PICK

Bootie Silicone Anal Plug. This anal plug is a mere 2 inches (5 centimeters) long, and has a soft, velvety texture. It's perfect for beginners who are interested in trying anal sex but want a bit of a warm-up first.

TOYS FOR HIM

Not all sex toys are made especially for women. Men can enjoy using toys in the bedroom, too. There are three basic categories of toys for men: male masturbators, prostate stimulators, and cock rings. Male masturbators are sleeves that are placed over the penis to simulate the sensations produced by vaginal sex and to bring him to orgasm. He uses his hand (or you can use yours) to move the sleeve up and down over his penis. Prostate stimulators are anal toys that are usually long, thin, and angled in a way that they can stimulate his prostate gland once they're inserted—and men who enjoy using them say they produce very intense orgasms. If your partner enjoys anal penetration, he might like these, too. Cock rings are rings made of silicone, rubber, or leather and can be placed at the base of the penis, or over the scrotum, to keep the blood that flows to the penis during arousal in the shaft. That means a longer erection. Some cock rings are solid, while others are snap-ons.

HOW TO USE IT

Once his penis is erect, you can slide a solid cock ring over it until the ring is in position at the base of his shaft. Or, if you have a snap-on version, you can fasten it around the base of the penis or around his scrotum.

BEST PICK

The Screaming O Vibrating Cock Ring. This inexpensive cock ring is a great starter for you and your partner. It's inexpensive, is textured with tiny knobs and "ticklers," and comes with a miniature motor, so it vibrates as well. That means if you use it during sex, it it can be equally as pleasurable for you as it is for him, because you'll get plenty of clitoral stimulation. And it's disposable, so if you find you're not that into it, you can just throw it away!

USING SEX TOYS SAFELY

Although using sex toys is generally safer than having sex with another person, it's still important to be aware of a few safety considerations. Some toys are made from more porous materials than others: if a toy is made from a porous material, like jelly rubber, PVC, or skin-like materials, bacteria can lodge in it, causing infections and disease transmission. Porous toys cannot be sterilized, making them risky if you're sharing them or simply with the passage of time. If you're using a porous toy, be sure to use a condom if it has ever been shared; if it's been used anally; or if you've had it for a long time. Nonporous toys, which are made of materials like silicone, steel, and glass, can easily be sterilized. You can boil them, or, in some cases, you can even put them in the dishwasher.

You should also be aware that some materials found in sex toys can actually be toxic. Because the production of sex toys isn't regulated in the United States, a company can easily label a product as "novelty use only"—which absolves the company of all responsibility if you use the toy as a sex toy. Some toys contain phthalates, which are chemical plasticizers that give some toys their squishy, bendy texture. Phthalates are carcinogens and have been banned in other parts of the world. So, to be on the safe side, avoid toys made from jelly rubber or PVC unless you are prepared to use them with condoms. And always steer clear of any toy that appears to be "weeping" or "sweating." Those are signs of chemical degradation, which happens when a product sits on a shelf for too long.

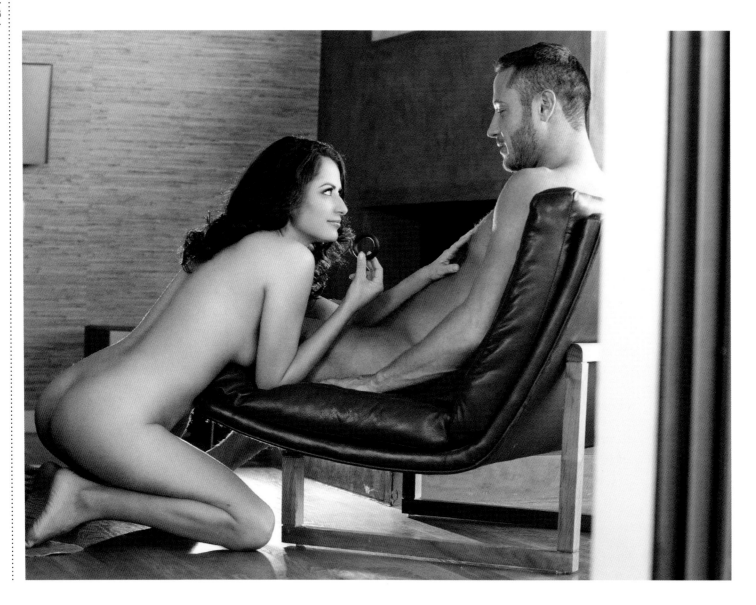

LUBRICANT

Because your arousal levels don't always correspond with your natural moisture levels, it's important to keep lubricant on hand. It's inexpensive, relatively easy to use, and can make your sex life more comfortable and pleasurable. Most lubricants can be bought in drugstores, but you can also find lubricant in some large chain stores, grocery stores, and sex shops. There are two basic types of lubricants: water-based and silicone-based. What's the difference? Here's a handy rundown on the pros and cons of each.

Water-Based Lubricant Pros

Absorbs into your body

Easy cleanup

Good for silicone-based sex toys

Condom compatible

Water-Based Lubricant Cons

Need to reapply often

May get dried out and sticky

Some contain glycerin, which can cause yeast infections, so check the label

Water-Based Lubricant Recommendations

Astroglide

Glycerin-Free Sticky Stuff

Silicone-Based Lubricant Pros

Lasts longer than water-based lubricants

Thinner texture

Can be used in water, so it's good for shower or bathtub use

Silicone-Based Lubricant Cons

Can damage silicone-based sex toys

Not absorbed by the body, so it must be washed off

Silicone-Based Lubricant Recommendations

Gun Oil Lubricant

Pink Lube

SEX TOY SHOPPING TIPS

In the past (and, in some places, in the present, too) buying a sex toy means making a trip to your local seedy sex shop, where you pray that no one notices you, avoid eye contact with other patrons, and then rush out with whatever you can grab and pay for quickly. But it doesn't have to be that way! In large cities like San Francisco, Los Angeles, and New York, progressive sex shops cater to women and couples, have educated staff, and provide a safe and comfortable environment for their customers to explore their options in toys and erotica. If your town doesn't have a sex shop along these lines, online shopping may be your best bet. Sex shops like Good Vibrations, The Pleasure Chest, and Toys in Babeland, for example, all have retail sites. They deliver items discreetly, feature how-to guides on their websites, and provide good customer service. If you are lucky enough to live near stores like these, take advantage of them: they often hold lectures, workshops, and training sessions on sexual practices and experiences that can help you explore your sexuality either on your own or as a couple. Before you go shopping, though, do some research online so you'll have a good idea of what you're looking for.

FEMINIST PORN

Pornography and other erotic media have been accused of everything from supporting sex addiction to exploiting women to causing sexism itself. The fact is, watching porn is an active choice, and it's your choice to make. Actually, everything about porn is a choice. The actors, directors, and producers choose to work in the industry, and the consumers choose to purchase it. Just be sure to make your choices wisely.

Many criticisms of porn tend to be one-sided. One complaint is that porn depicts women as sex objects. The truth is there's a wide range of porn on the market, and while some porn does objectify women, it also objectifies men. Most pornography shows the man's penis only, with very few shots of his face or the rest of his body. In porn like this, men are portrayed as constantly erect sex robots, while women always seem to be young and oversexed. But not all porn is created equal.

Today, there's a wide range of porn that's being created by women and for women—and there's even a feminist porn movement. According to the authors of *The Feminist Porn Book* (2012), feminist porn is a genre that uses "sexually explicit imagery to contest and complicate dominant representations of gender, sexuality, race, ethnicity, class, ability, age, body type, and other identity markers." Feminist porn is anything but traditional: it "seeks to unsettle conventional definitions of sex, and expand the language of sex as an erotic activity, an expression of identity, a power exchange, a cultural commodity, and even as new politics." It also seeks to support fair treatment of the actors on-set, and to depict a range of sexualities. Don't be fooled—none of this means that feminist porn, or any porn that's geared toward women, has to be soft, gentle, and romantic. While some women do enjoy this type of sexual scenario, others are turned on by watching power exchanges or taboo scenarios. It's up to you to explore erotica for yourself, and to discover what gets you hot and bothered.

PORN'S PLUSES

Jackie Strano is vice president of Good Vibrations, a San Francisco–based sex corporation that's sex-positive and woman-run. Here's what she has to say about porn: "Any relationship ruined by porn-watching needed help to begin with. Porn can help enhance fantasy play, teach old dogs new tricks, and help kick arousal into overdrive. That's due to porn's visual stimulation, especially when it comes to scenes that are often the subject of fantasies. The naughty factor can be fun and thrilling. Honestly, some folks get most of their sex education from porn, so that's why we love to showcase explicit movies that show couples communicating about sex, using lube and barriers when needed, having fun—*and* having real orgasms!"

SEVEN REASONS WHY PORN IS GOOD FOR YOU

Porn can benefit you by:

1. Teaching you a thing or two. Porn can teach you new sexual skills and behaviors, from sexual positions to step-by-step how-tos. Watching someone perform an act you'd like to try helps you understand the dynamics and mechanics of the movement.

2. Letting you explore in a safe environment. Whether you want to learn a few new tricks by watching porn or you're just feeling frisky, porn lets you explore sexual options in the safety of your own bedroom before you try them with a partner. You decide whether you want to watch porn alone or with a partner—and you don't have to worry about safety or being judged.

3. Inspiring fantasies. Watching erotic films can open your mind and expose you to sexual scenarios you might not have considered otherwise. Lots of these ideas will be fantasies— great for calling to mind when you're masturbating— but you might want to make some of them happen with your partner.

4. Showing you what "real" sex looks like. Gone are the days when your only porn options involved surgically enhanced women faking orgasms. Feminist porn, alt porn, and amateur porn all show real women having real orgasms. Seeing a range of body types and sex acts demonstrates that sexuality is not one-dimensional but multifaceted.

5. Cluing you in on new ways to masturbate. Lots of female erotica, like how-to guides or erotic films, show women masturbating. This can give you exciting new ideas for positions, methods, speed, and intensity.

6. Showcasing shiny new toys. Porn films often show sex toys in action. Watch porn with your partner to explore what looks good to both of you—and what you might like to try together.

7. Opening a dialogue. Watching porn with your partner can actually bring you closer together. It's an easy way to start a sexual dialogue about what you like, what you'd like to do more of, and how you want to experiment.

Remember, porn can be great for inspiration or watching a particular act before deciding whether to try it yourself. While there is more quality porn available than in recent years, please understand that porn is not always accurate and risky behavior may be portrayed, such as anal sex without lubricant, group sex without condoms, or jumping right into penetration without foreplay. Don't translate what you see in porn verbatim to your sex life. Educate yourself about sexual safety and use your common sense.

Knowing what's available in terms of sex toys and erotica means it'll be easier for you to make a conscious, educated choice—and be satisfied with what you buy. Relax and experiment, either solo or with your partner—it's the best way to find out what gets you off and what satisfies you. Read on to find out how to add a dash of kink to your sex life.

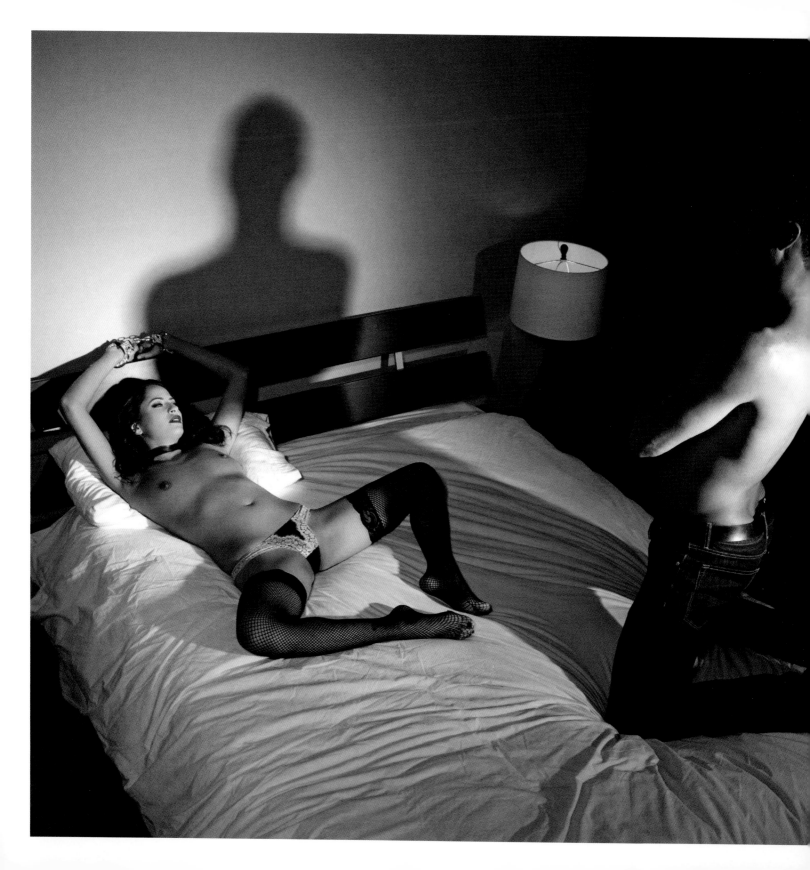

11

Alternative Lifestyles and Practices: Threesomes, BDSM, and Lots More

It's deceptively easy to think of sexuality in terms of polar opposites—that is, straight or gay. The truth is, though, that sexuality comprises a wide spectrum or continuum, as sexologist Alfred Kinsey argued in his groundbreaking 1948 article, "Sexual Behavior of the Human Male." Kinsey's spectrum focused on sexual orientation, but the same idea can be applied to sex practices in general.

There's no such thing as "absolutely right" or "absolutely wrong" when it comes to sex as long as it takes place between consenting adults, so when it comes to experimenting with alternative lifestyles, it's up to you to set your own priorities and limits. If you're single, alternative sex practices can be a fun way for you to explore and discover new dimensions of your sexuality; if you're part of a couple, they can strengthen your relationship with your partner and make your love life seriously adventurous. Sound interesting? Keep reading: this chapter will show you how to experiment safely with threesomes; swinging; bondage, discipline, sadism, and masochism (BDSM); and much more.

THE SEXUAL ORIENTATION CONTINUUM

We've established that sexual orientation isn't as simple as black or white. It exists on a continuum, with heterosexuality on one end and homosexuality on the other, and most people find that their personal sexual orientation lies somewhere between these two extremes. What's more, it's likely that your sexual identification will change over the course of your life. That means your sexual orientation isn't fixed: it's fluid. While Kinsey was conducting his pioneering sex research in the 1950s, he found that between 6% and 14% of women reported that they'd had at least an incidental sexual experience with another woman. Today, it's likely that those figures are much higher (and plus, it's important to remember that statistics in sexual research are typically higher than reported due to the stigma that's attached to talking about sex in many Western cultures).

What this means for you is that it's perfectly normal to experiment with women, even if you consider yourself "straight." Women who enjoy being sexual with other women often feel that it's a very different experience from being with a man: our bodies tend to feel softer to the touch than men's; women may be more in tune with each other's emotions; and they might be more likely to understand another woman's body and sexual needs. Maybe you want to experiment with being with a woman on your own, or maybe you're interested in having a threesome with your partner. Feel free to play within your comfort zone, whether you identify as heterosexual, heteroflexible, bisexual, homosexual, or somewhere in between.

NONMONOGAMY: THREESOMES, SWINGING, AND POLYAMORY

Monogamy is, simply, the choice to be sexually exclusive with one partner. A relationship is nonmonogamous when the two individuals involved choose to open their sexual relationship to include other people. That's not to say it's easy to choose nonmonogamy, though. Both you and your partner need to consider the benefits and risks carefully, to respect each other's boundaries, and, most of all, to communicate well. While it's not for everyone, couples who manage nonmonogamy well through great communication effectively eliminate the possibility of having affairs or cheating, because they've already agreed to have sex with other partners. The three most common types of nonmonogamy are threesomes, swinging, and polyamory.

THREESOMES

Fantasizing about a threesome is really common—but it's up to you to choose whether you want to turn that fantasy into reality. A threesome can be exciting and arousing, but it may damage your relationship unless you and your partner are explicit about the rules and boundaries that are acceptable to you both. After a threesome, it's possible that one or more of the people involved might experience feelings of jealousy and insecurity. Do your best to prevent this in advance. Sit down with your partner and talk about all the details. Use these five questions as guidelines:

1. Who will the third person in your threesome be? Male or female? Will he or she be a friend, or someone you connect with on a dating site?

2. How will you initiate things? Will it start as a date, with dinner and drinks, or would you rather get right to the point and straight into bed?

3. Talk about the specifics of the interaction. If the third person is female, is he allowed to penetrate her? Touch her? Kiss her?

4. What will happen when he is ready to ejaculate? Is he allowed to finish in, or on, the new partner?

5. What will happen afterward? Will the new partner leave? Stay overnight? Will either of you contact the new partner in the future for friendly or sexual interactions?

Having this conversation not only helps you establish clear, defined boundaries, but it also forces you to view the situation through a more realistic lens. Be perceptive about your own needs: if you start to feel uncomfortable or jealous while talking to your partner about the rules of the threesome, this may not be the right time for you to try it. And that's fine—sometimes just talking about a threesome can be a massive turn-on. Many couples enjoy the "tease" of the idea of a threesome without actually engaging in one. If you and your partner are one of these couples, make sure he's clear that it's just a fantasy before he brings a new friend home. The idea of a threesome might be more exciting than the actual experience.

If you're comfortable discussing the rules of the threesome with your partner and you're ready take it to the next level, be mindful of the following before you get your ménage à trois on. *First, stay busy and attentive.* If your triad turns into a duo, one person might feel ignored and awkward. Be sure to be generous with both of your partners. *Second, stay safe.* Even if you usually enjoy condom-free sex with your monogamous partner, you'll still need to use precautions and protection when having a threesome. If he penetrates both of you, be sure to change the condom before he switches partners. You might also want to consider using a dental dam or protective latex barrier when having oral sex with a new partner.

OPEN RELATIONSHIPS, SWINGING, AND POLYAMORY

Swinging is a sex act in which monogamous partners have sex with other individuals or couples for pleasure and fun, but not for the purpose of creating an intimate relationship. It's easy for swingers to find like-minded people on the Internet, where lots of local swingers' groups have websites—some of which have as many as 100,000 members. Swingers' events can take place in each other's homes or at a private club. Just like having a threesome, the choice to swing, or to bring other people sexually into your relationship in any way, requires two vital things: communication and comfort. Both parties must be happy with the decision, and it's important to set boundaries. If you're thinking of swinging with your partner, review the earlier questions for threesomes: they'll help you decide whether you're ready.

Polyamory is consensual, ethical, and responsible nonmonogamy. Polyamorous couples—often referred to as poly couples—agree to seek out intimate relationships outside of their primary relationship. Poly couples feel that monogamy isn't necessary for a healthy, bonded, intimate partnership. While these other relationships may be sexual, polyamory isn't purely based on sexuality or sex acts. Successful poly couples need to have exceptional communication skills—and they often do. That helps them set strict boundaries when it comes to building new relationships, and how those relationships will affect their primary relationship. Each couple creates their own set of rules and boundaries. Some couples date a third person together; in other couples, only one partner is permitted to pursue an outside relationship. Still other couples develop relationships with other couples. While there are benefits to polyamory, such as more sex, affection, and variety, challenges—such as jealousy—do exist. So how do poly couples make it work? Top-notch communication and negotiation skills.

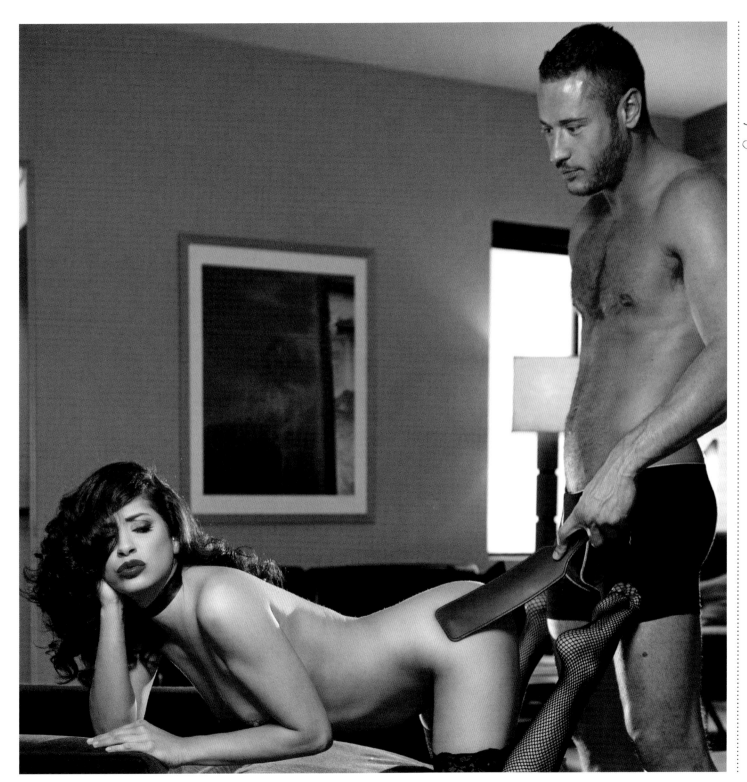

ADVICE FROM A POLYAMOROUS WIFE: JENNIFER'S PERSPECTIVE

Robert, forty-five, and Jennifer, thirty-eight, are a successful, educated, and happily married couple of twenty years. They are also polyamorous, and have been from the beginning of their relationship. Here's what Jennifer has to say about:

The terms and boundaries of their relationship: "The terms and boundaries of our relationship are fluid and change based on the situation and the moment, as well as what's going on in our lives at that time. However, under our current terms, we operate as a team. We seek polyamorous relationships as a team. When you get us, you get us both. It tends to make things a bit more complex in some ways—but more stable in other ways."

Challenges and boundary violations: "One of the biggest challenges has been our intensity of feelings toward new partners. We were involved in a long-term triad relationship—a complex dynamic that, in the end, meant that not everyone was on the same page in terms of the goals of the relationship, and not everyone felt the same level of connection. It's a lot to coordinate, and it's complicated, to say the least! Ultimately, we ended that relationship because we realized that it just wasn't going to fit with our primary goals. Like I said, our current rule is that we operate as a team. Violating that rule means *not* operating as a team! And that's happened, too. Essentially, one of us—usually me—decided to hook up with someone

while the other wasn't present. Again, depending on the individual experience, this might have been okay—or it definitely might *not* have been okay—in which case, we handled it with much discussion, reassessment, and trust-building."

Benefits to being polyamorous: "It's a lot of fun to be who you are, and to accept that we have sexual attractions to more than one person. It's not even realistic to think that we *wouldn't* be attracted to other people. It's repressive to deny these feelings, and I think monogamy is a soul-crushing disappointment to many people. Having a loving, long-term relationship with someone shouldn't have to mean narrowing the scope of your sexuality. I love that I can experience other people sexually. When they're executed in the spirit of our 'team' relationship, these outside experiences only enhance our own relationship, and bring us closer together. Furthermore, loving other people is really beautiful, and it makes life so rich. We have huge capacities for love—whether it lasts for a moment or a lifetime."

Advice to monogamous couples: "Talk about everything. Talk about the stuff that feels uncomfortable and hard to navigate. Then navigate it together. Never stop talking. Listen to your instincts, and don't deny your feelings. If something feels bad, stop, talk, and work through it."

50 SHADES OF KINK: BDSM AND FETISH

With the presence of some aspects of fetish and bondage in pop culture and the media, more and more people are curious about BDSM. There are some benefits to the fact that these previously underground practices are becoming more mainstream, including safer spaces for sexual experimentation and increased acceptance for people who make them part of their lifestyles. BDSM is a general term for practices that involve a variety of behaviors, including role play, bondage, restraint, and power dynamics. They often involve one "dominant" partner and one "submissive" partner who have negotiated the limits and boundaries of the experience in advance. Regardless of the scenario, it's vital that both parties trust and respect each other. The BDSM community uses the phrase "safe, sane, and consensual," or SSC, to describe the way BDSM experiences should be played out.

Individual responsibility is also a big part of the BDSM experience. Members of the community stick to the motto RACK—that is, risk-aware consensual kink. That means it's up to each person to be aware of the risks inherent in the practices he or she engages in. BDSM activities run the gamut from "light," such as role play or spanking, to "heavy," such as extreme bondage; sexual intercourse may or may not occur within BDSM play. As with all other sex acts, it's important to be mindful of your partner at all times, and to establish a safety word beforehand to let your partner know when you really need to stop the play.

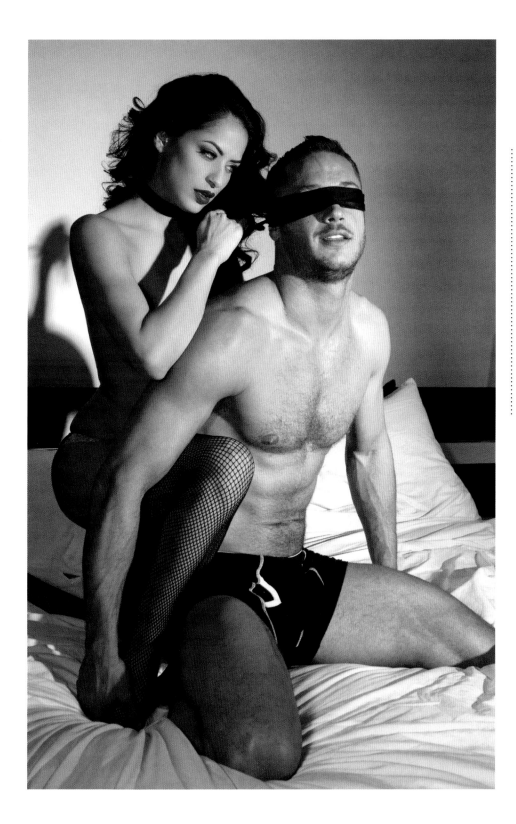

FETISH ADVICE FROM MODEL ULORIN VEX

"I strongly believe in the importance of communication, always; in not being afraid to experiment; and in telling your partner what you'd like to explore. Most of my kinky friends and I have learned to be very open and honest: it's so refreshing. If you're new to kink, start out light. For instance, start with playful spanking before you try hardcore flogging. That'll let you find out what you enjoy and what you don't. And of course, be aware that consent—meaning explicit, informed verbal approval—is of the utmost importance."

The world of BDSM uses lots of tools and toys. Here's a BDSM toolbox for your own bedroom. Always be sure to ask your partner in advance for his consent before you start the action.

Whip or flogger. This is typically a piece of leather, or multiple pieces, that strike the skin. Using a tool to strike the skin places the whip-wielder in a position of power, and can excite and stimulate the other partner. Try this: have the partner on the receiving end bend over, get down on all fours, or stand against the wall with hands at his or her sides or above the head. The "whipper" can start by lightly drawing the whip or flog over the receiver's bottom, being careful not to let the device hit the back or legs.

Crop. A crop is a stiff striking device used for discipline by spanking, striking, and other sensory activities. (When using for spanking, make sure the end of the crop with a stiff piece of leather is far enough away from the buttocks that it doesn't wrap around and snap on your partner.) As you would with a whip or flogger, have your partner bend over or stand against the wall with his arms out to the side or above his head. Use the middle part of the crop to spank his bottom. Run the top part around his buttocks, back, legs, and even genitals (carefully and softly) for a light, teasing sensation.

Handcuffs or wrist restraints. Handcuffs and restraints can be used to keep your partner from moving or to limit his movement while you have your wicked (or not-so-wicked) way with him. Try restraining your partner while you perform oral sex on him, or, better yet, have him perform it on you.

Blindfolds. These can demonstrate psychological submission and create sensory deprivation. They can be lots of fun during both foreplay and intercourse. Restrict your partner's vision with the blindfold, then kiss and stroke your partner's body. Slowly move closer to his sexual parts, and watch how your partner reacts to the sensations.

Full-body restraints. A set of full-body restraints can be used for a more intense, full-body bondage experience that takes movement restriction to a whole new level. Requirements? A very trusting relationship with your partner, and a good bit of practice. Typically, full-body restraints are made to be attached to the four corners of your bed.

BEGINNER BDSM BASICS

Start with verbal play. Verbalizing a power dynamic is not only a great start to BDSM, but it can also be really exciting for your partner. Before you start, talk to your partner and tell each other which words turn you on—and off. For example, some couples like to use more explicit talk, such as *pussy* or *fuck me*, while other prefer "textbook" terms, like *penis*, *vagina*, or *sex*. Use your favorite kind of dirty talk to take control, and tell him what you want him to do to you. Have fun bossing him around in bed! If he's into it, have him be the power bottom—that's someone who aggressively prefers to be the recipient or submissive party in an act. You can also use language that implies power roles. For example, you can have him refer to you as a goddess, mistress, or madam, while you refer to him as the slave.

Grab a blindfold and tie it loosely around his head. Have him sit or lie on the bed. Deprived of his visual capacities, his other senses will be heightened. Use this to your advantage. Treat his skin to new sensations by running ice or warm candle wax over it. Whisper in his ear and let your breath tickle him. Feed him sweet, delicious, richly-textured foods, like chocolate, ice cream, or fruit. When you're ready, remove the blindfold, and take advantage of his state of arousal.

Dress the part by wearing fetishized clothing like stockings or corsets, or try role-play costumes such as secretary, nurse, or schoolgirl. Act out a character based on your outfit. Or try leaving your heels or boots on while you take off everything else. That'll be enough to make you feel like a sex bomb! You'll feel hot and kinky in your get-up, while he'll go crazy over the visuals. Experiment with tying each other up, using rope, restraints, or handcuffs. While you're restrained, have your partner start pleasuring you with gentle, loving kisses, light bites, and soft spankings—and proceed from there. Being at the mercy of your partner and giving up all control over the situation is an arousing act of trust.

Whether you want to try out a threesome, experiment with swinging, or get tied down or dressed up, adding a little kink to your sexual routine can be an exciting and adventurous way to keep things hot in the bedroom. Go on, get creative. As long as you and your partner set boundaries and respect them, there's nothing you shouldn't try.

TOP 5 FILMS FEATURING BDSM AND FETISH

1. *The Secretary* (1995). In this film, a young woman who is naturally submissive gains employment as a secretary and plays out her tendencies with her boss. Even though she is submissive, she finds empowerment through the sexual play. Themes include BDSM, restraining, equestrian fetish, and overall powerplay.

2. *Eyes Wide Shut* (1999). This erotic thriller depicts the tension between a married couple and explores a variety of uncomfortable or taboo sexual situations. Over the space of a few days, the protagonist undergoes temptations to his marriage—including being hired to perform at a sex orgy with masked individuals in a secret society.

3. *The Story of O* (1975). The main character is taken to a retreat by her boyfriend, where she's subjected to sexual perversions and is trained in bondage and discipline.

4. *9½ Weeks* (1986). This film chronicles a love affair that includes a variety of BDSM and kink-related themes, such as blindfolds, power exchange, public sex, and gender fluidity.

5. *Caligula* (1979). This erotic historical film depicts the sexual experiences of Caligula as he makes his way to the throne. This film, which explores themes such as group sex, was also released with hardcore inserts that leave nothing to the imagination.

Resources

FEMALE ISSUES/ FEMINISM

The Second Sex by Simone de Beauvoir

The Vagina Monologues by Eve Ensler

The Feminine Mystique by Betty Friedan

Female Chauvinist Pigs by Ariel Levy

Our Bodies, Ourselves by The Boston Women's Health Collective

Revolution from Within: A Book of Self-Esteem by Gloria Steinem

BITCHfest: Ten Years of Cultural Criticism from the Pages of Bitch Magazine by Danya Ruttenberg

Women: An Intimate Geography by Natalie Angier

WEBSITES

www.feministpress.org

www.feminist.org

www.now.org

SUPPORT GROUPS

Visit www.psychologytoday.com and search for your local support groups.

ANATOMY AND SEXUALITY

Our Bodies, Ourselves by The Boston Women's Collective

The Joy of Sex by Alex Comfort

Guide to Getting It On! A Book About the Wonders of Sex by Paul Joannides and Gröss Daerick Sr.

Nina Hartley's Guide to Total Sex by Nina Hartley

Dr. Sprinkle's Spectacular Sex: Make Over Your Love Life with One of the World's Great Sex Experts by Annie Sprinkle

G-SPOT

The G-Spot: And Other Discoveries about Human Sexuality by Alice Khan Ladas, Beverly Whipple, and John D. Perry

Clit-ology: Master Every Move from A to G-Spot to Give Her Ultimate Pleasure by Jordan LaRousse and Samantha Sade

The Clitoral Truth: The Secret World at Your Fingertips by Rebecca Chalker

Smart Girl's Guide to the G-Spot by Violet Blue

The Secrets of Great G-Spot Orgasms and Female Ejaculations by Tristan Taormino

ORGASM

I Love Female Orgasm: An Extraordinary Orgasm Guide by Dorian Solot, Marshall Miller, and Shirley Chiang

The Science of Orgasm by Barry R. Komisaruk, Carlos Beyer-Flores, and Beverly Whipple

The Ultimate Guide to Orgasm for Women: How to Become Orgasmic for a Lifetime by Mikaya Heart and Violet Blue

REPRODUCTIVE INFORMATION AND BIRTH CONTROL

Woman of Valor: Margaret Sanger and the Birth Control Movement in America by Ellen Chesler

www.ourbodiesourselves.org

www.plannedparenthood.org

PREGNANCY AND POSTPARTUM SEX

Your Orgasmic Pregnancy: Little Sex Secrets Every Hot Mama Should Know (Positively Sexual) by Danielle Cavallucci and Yvonne K. Fulbright

SEX AND MENOPAUSE

Harvard Medical School: Sexuality in Midlife and Beyond by Jan Leslie Shifren, et al.

The Sex Bible for People Over 50 by Laurie Betito

Naked at Our Age by Joan Price

WEBSITES

www.ourbodiesourselves.org

MASTURBATION

Getting Off: A Woman's Guide to Masturbation by Jamye Waxman

Sex for One by Betty Dodson

MARRIAGE

Passionate Marriage by Dr. David Schnarch

Partners in Passion: A Guide to Great Sex, Emotional Intimacy and Long-term Love by Mark Michaels and Patricia Johnson

Mating in Captivity: Reconciling the Erotic and the Domestic by Esther Perel

PORN

The Feminist Porn Book by Tristan Taormino, Constance Penley, Celine Parrenas Shimizu, and Mireille Miller-Young

The Smart Girl's Guide to Porn by Violet Blue

DANCE AND MOVEMENT

The S Factor: Strip Workouts for Every Woman by Sheila Kelly

Burlesque and the Art of the Teese by Dita Von Teese and Bronwyn Garrity

Fetish and the Art of the Teese by Dita Von Teese and Bronwyn Garrity

ANAL

The Anal Sex Position Guide by Tristan Taormino

ORAL SEX

Oral Sex You'll Never Forget by Sonia Borg

The Art of Oral Sex by Ian Denchasy and Alicia Denchasy

KINK/BDSM

Whipping Girl: A Transsexual Woman on Sexism and the Scapegoating of Femininity by Julia Serano

The Little Book of Kink by Dr. Jessica O'Reilly

The Sexually Dominant Woman by Lady Green

Screw the Roses, Send Me the Thorns by Phillip Miller and Molly Devon

The Seductive Art of Japanese Bondage by Midori

The Ultimate Guide to Kink: BDSM, Role Play, and the Erotic Edge by Tristan Taormino

SEX TOYS

The Big Book of Sex Toys by Tristan Taormino

Toygasms: The Insider's Guide to Sex Toys by Dr. Sadie Allison

Good Vibrations: New Complete Guide to Vibrators by Joani Blank with Ann Whidden

WEBSITES

www.ThePleasureChest.com

www.Babeland.com

www.GoodVibes.com

OPEN RELATIONSHIPS/ POLYAMORY

The Ethical Slut: A Practical Guide to Polyamory, Open Relationships & Other Adventures by Dossie Easton and Janet W. Hardy

Opening Up by Tristan Taormino

WEBSITES

www.polychromatic.com

INSPIRATION FROM LITERATURE

Lysistrata by Aristophanes

The Story of O by Pauline Reage

Lust: Erotic Fantasies for Women by Violet Blue

OTHER

Erotic Massage by Charla Hathaway

Index

adrenaline, 76
AIDS. *See* HIV/AIDS.
alternative lifestyles
    BDSM, 180, 181, 182–183
    nonmonogamy, 177, 178
    polyamory, 178, 180
    sexual orientation, 176
    swinging, 178
    threesomes, 177–178
anal play
    bacteria and, 147
    blow jobs and, 144, 147, 154
    Bootie Silicone Anal Plug, 168
    communication and, 139, 142
    condoms and, 147
    dental dams and, 137, 139, 154
    double penetration, 142–143, 146
    external mouth play, 137, 139, 154
    fecal matter and, 139
    history of, 135
    hygiene and, 147
    Kegel exercises and, 147
    light penetration, 139
    lubrication and, 139, 142, 168
    Man on Top position, 143
    men and, 144, 154
    nonpenetrative finger play, 137
    oral sex and, 137, 144, 147, 154
    orgasms and, 146
    over the clothes, 137
    pegging, 144
    penetration, 142–144
    physical reactions to, 146, 147
    pleasurability of, 137
    porn and, 136, 146, 147
    pregnancy and, 39
    preparing for, 139, 142
    prevalence of, 136
    psychological pleasurability of, 137
    Rear Entry position, 144
    relaxation and, 139, 142, 146
    risks of, 147
    safety precautions, 147
    sex toys and, 139, 144, 165, 168
    Spooning position, 143
    Woman on Top position, 144
Angel, Joanna, 154
attraction, 80

bacterial vaginosis (BV), 28
Bartholin's glands, 19
BDSM, 180, 181, 182–183
behavioral birth control, 25
Better Sex video series, 60
birth control. *See also* condoms; pregnancy.

barrier methods, 25
behavioral methods, 25
education on, 24
forties and, 48
hormonal methods, 25
intrauterine devices (IUDs), 25
ovulation and, 95
postpartum, 41
bisexuality, 82, 176
blended orgasms, 91, 92, 164
blow jobs. *See also* male body; oral sex.
    anal play and, 144, 147, 154
    anxiety and, 150
    breasts and, 152
    communication and, 150–151, 154, 157
    condoms and, 160
    creativity with, 152
    deep throating, 155
    ejaculation and, 155
    empowerment of, 150
    exhaustion and, 152, 153
    full-body experience, 157
    glans and, 100
    hands with, 150–151
    hand-to-mouth transition, 151
    pace of, 152
    perineum and, 154
    safety, 160
    69 position, 160
    spitting vs. swallowing, 105
    STIs and, 105
    teasing, 150–151
    testicles and, 154
    view and, 150
Bootie Silicone Anal Plug, 168
brain. *See also* oxytocin.
    adrenaline, 76
    attraction chemistry, 80
    committed love and, 77, 80
    dopamine, 74
    estrogen, 76
    gender differences, 80, 82
    hypothalamus, 73, 82
    imprinting, 80
    intimacy and, 77, 80, 82
    lust and, 77, 80
    neuroplasticity, 72, 73
    neurotransmitters, 71, 72, 73, 74, 77
    nitric oxide, 76
    parasympathetic relaxation, 76
    phenylethylamine, 77
    pheromones and, 80
    prolactin, 76
    serotonin, 74, 76
    testosterone, 76
    triangular theory of love, 77
    vasopressin, 75, 76
breasts
    age and, 15

areolas, 14
blow jobs and, 152
communication and, 17
examination of, 17
familiarization with, 17
lactation, 14
milk glands, 14
nipples, 14, 15, 17
pregnancy and, 14
ptosis, 15
resolution phase and, 88
self-image and, 16
sizes, 15, 16
stimulation and, 17

Caligula (film), 183
car sex, 133
casual sex, 38, 45, 49, 56, 57, 68
cervix, 20, 39, 88
Charm Silicone Dildo, 167
chlamydia, 28, 38, 105, 160
circumcision, 100
clitoris. *See also* external sex organs.
    cunnilingus and, 157
    erection of, 19
    glans, 18
    location of, 18
    masturbation and, 65
    orgasms and, 86, 91, 95
    positions and, 114, 126, 143
    sex toys and, 164, 165
    Spooning position and, 143
    Thigh Master position and, 126
clothing, 137, 183
cock rings, 169
communication
    anal play and, 139, 142
    BDSM and, 180, 182
    blow jobs and, 150–151, 154, 157
    breasts and, 17
    confidence and, 60
    cunnilingus and, 158, 159
    erectile disfunction (ED) and, 111
    hand jobs and, 107
    masturbation as, 87
    orgasms and, 87
    polyamory and, 180
    porn and, 173
    postpartum sex and, 40
    pregnancy and, 39
    sex toys and, 166
    sexual self-esteem and, 60, 68
    STIs and, 68
    threesomes and, 177
    tips for, 62
condoms. *See also* birth control.
    anal play and, 147
    as birth control, 25, 41
    blow jobs and, 160

buying, 24
health and, 24
lubrication and, 171
open relationships and, 39
porn and, 173
postpartum sex and, 41
sex toys and, 139, 165, 169
shower sex and, 130
STIs and, 24, 28, 29, 38, 39, 50
threesomes and, 178
usage guide, 27
corona, 100
corpora cavernosa, 100
corpus spongiosum, 100
cortisol, 45
"Cowgirl" position. *See* Woman on Top position.
Cowper's glands, 103, 106
cunnilingus. *See also* oral sex.
bathing and, 158
clitoris and, 157
communication and, 158, 159
confidence and, 157
dental dams and, 160, 178
lubrication and, 158
positions for, 160
safety, 160, 178
self-exploration and, 158
shaving/waxing and, 158
69 position, 160
STIs and, 160
cyclic guanosine monophosphate (cGMP), 111

Davidson, Richard, 72
dental dams
anal play and, 137, 139, 154
cunnilingus and, 160, 178
STIs and, 25
threesomes and, 178
dildos, 167, 168
divorce, 49
dopamine, 74
douching, 24
dyspareunia, 97

ejaculation
blow jobs and, 155
female, 22, 94
male, 103, 104, 110
preejaculatory fluid, 25, 103, 105, 106
semen and, 104–105, 106, 155
epinephrine. *See* adrenaline.
erectile dysfunction (ED), 110
erections, 100, 106, 107
estrogen
birth control and, 25, 41
menstruation and, 95
ovaries and, 20
overview of, 76
perimenopause and, 45

prolapse and, 50
vaginal dryness and, 48, 52
exercise, 59
experimentation, 38
external sex organs. *See also* clitoris.
Bartholin's glands, 19
glans, 18
hymen, 19
introitus, 19
labia majora, 18, 88, 158
mons, 18
prepuce, 18
urinary meatus, 18, 19
Eyes Wide Shut (film), 183

fallopian tubes, 20
fatalemedia.com, 144
female ejaculation, 22, 94
Feminist Porn Book, The, 172
fertility awareness, 25
fifties, sex in, 49–50
Fisher, Helen, 72
Fonda, Jane, 52
foreplay
blindfolds and, 182
brain and, 73
breasts and, 17
fifties and, 50
hand jobs, 107
multiple orgasms and, 92
orgasms and, 92, 95
plateau phase and, 88
premature ejaculation and, 110
shower and, 130
foreskin, 100
forties, sex in, 43–45, 48–49
frenulum, 100, 108
fundus, 20

genital herpes, 29, 105, 160
glans
female, 18
male, 100
gonorrhea, 28, 38, 105, 160
Good Vibrations corporation, 144, 167, 171, 172
G-spot. *See also* internal sex organs.
ejaculation and, 22
female ejaculation and, 94
location of, 22
male, 103
Man on Top position, 116
masturbation and, 65
orgasms and, 91, 95, 97
Pinwheel position, 121
positions for, 116, 121
purpose of, 22
Rear Entry position, 118, 144
sex toys and, 165, 167

Sitting position, 121
stimulating, 22
gynecological exams, 24

hand jobs, 107–108, 110
Handstand Rear Entry position, 124
hepatitis A/B/C, 29, 105
herpes. *See* genital herpes.
Hitachi Magic Wand, 165
HIV/AIDS, 29, 105, 147
homosexuality, 135, 176
hormonal birth control, 25
human papilloma virus (HPV), 29, 160
hymen, 19
hypothalamus, 73, 82

imprinting, 80
internal sex organs. *See also* G-spot.
cervix, 20, 39, 88
fallopian tubes, 20
fundus, 20
isthmus, 20
myometrium, 20
ovaries, 20
perimetrium, 20
Skene's glands, 94
uterus, 20, 39, 88
intrauterine devices (IUDs), 25
introitus, 19
isthmus, 20

Johnson, Virginia, 20, 88, 92, 106, 117
Journal of Sex Research, 110–111
journals, 10, 59

Kegel exercises, 43, 45, 48, 94, 147
Kinsey, Alfred, 175, 177

labia majora, 18, 88, 158
lubrication
anal play and, 139, 142, 168
Bartholin's glands and, 19
cunnilingus and, 158
dildos and, 167
estrogen and, 48
perimenopause and, 45
selecting, 48
sex toys and, 168
shower sex and, 130
types of, 171

male body. *See also* blow jobs.
anal play and, 144, 154
ejaculation, 103, 104, 106–107
ejaculation issues, 110
emotional issues, 110–111
erectile dysfunction (ED), 110
hand jobs, 107–108, 110
penis, 100, 103

plateau phase, 106
preejaculatory fluid, 25, 103, 105, 106
premature ejaculation, 110
P-spot, 103
refractory period, 107
resolution phase, 107
scrotum, 100
semen, 104–105
seminal vesicles, 103
seminiferous tubules, 103
sex toys and, 165, 166, 169
sexual response, 106–107
sperm, 25, 27, 100, 103
testicles, 100, 103, 106, 108
vas deferens, 103
Viagra, 111
Man on Top position, 115–116, 133, 143
Masters, William, 20, 88, 92, 106, 117
masturbation
    ambiance and, 61
    benefits of, 61
    clitoral stimulation, 65
    communication as, 87
    G-spot and, 65
    learning and, 36
    mental preparation for, 64
    orgasms and, 95
    porn and, 173
    positions for, 64
    postpartum sex and, 43
    prevalence of, 61
    seventies and, 52
    sex toys and, 65
    techniques, 65
meditation, 10
menopause, 45, 50, 52
menstruation
    endometrium and, 20
    forties and, 48
    orgasms and, 95
    puberty and, 34
    "rhythm" method and, 25
Missionary Style position. See Man on Top position.
Modified Missionary with Elevated Hips position, 97
mons, 18
multiple orgasms, 92
myometrium, 20

neuroplasticity, 72, 73
neurotransmitters, 71, 72, 73, 74, 77
9½ Weeks (film), 183
nitric oxide, 76
nonmonogamy, 177, 178

oral sex. See also blow jobs; cunnilingus.
    anal play and, 137, 144, 147
    dental dams, 160, 178
    full-body experience, 157
    pregnancy and, 39
    teeth brushing and, 105
orgasms

anal play and, 146
biological issues, 97
blended orgasms, 91, 92, 164
clitoral, 86, 91, 95
comfort with partner and, 95
communication and, 87
dyspareunia and, 97
"ejaculatory inevitability," 106
excitement phase, 88
faking, 87
female ejaculation, 94
G-spot and, 91, 95, 97
increasing frequency of, 95
increasing intensity of, 95
infrequency of, 86
lack of, 11, 86, 97
male, 103, 104, 106–107
masturbation and, 95
medical attention for, 97
medical issues and, 97
menstruation and, 95
Modified Missionary with Elevated Hips position, 97
mood and, 95
multiple orgasms, 92
multiple stimulation and, 95
myths, 86
orgasm phase, 88
oxytocin and, 75
plateau phase, 88, 106
pregnancy and, 43
psychological issues and, 97
Rear Entry position, 97
refractory period, 107
resolution phase, 88, 107
sex toys and, 164
vaginal orgasms, 91
vaginismus and, 97
Woman on Top position, 97
ovaries, 20
oxytocin. See also brain.
    bonding and, 14, 44, 73, 74–75, 76
    gender differences with, 82
    lactation and, 14
    postpartum sex and, 40, 44–45
    production of, 74–75, 76

parasympathetic relaxation, 76
Peepshow position, 122
pelvic floor, 45, 48
penis
    circumcision, 100
    corona, 100
    corpora cavernosa, 100
    corpus spongiosum, 100
    Cowper's glands, 103, 106
    cyclic guanosine monophosphate (cGMP), 111
    erectile dysfunction (ED), 110
    erections, 100, 106, 107
    foreskin, 100
    frenulum, 100, 108
    glans, 100

shaft, 100
sizes of, 103
urethra, 100, 103, 106
perimenopause, 45, 48
perimetrium, 20
phenylethylamine, 77
pheromones, 80
Pick-Me-Up position, 127
Pinwheel position, 121
plastic surgery, 67
Pleasure Chest, The website, 171
polyamory, 178, 180
porn
    anal play and, 136, 146, 147
    benefits of, 173
    communication and, 173
    education and, 60
    feminist porn, 172
    masturbation and, 61, 173
    sex toys and, 173
positions
    anal play and, 142–144
    bed positions, 129
    car positions, 133
    chair positions, 132–133
    clitoris and, 114
    couch positions, 132–133
    cunnilingus and, 160
    deep-throating and, 155
    female ejaculation and, 94
    G-spot and, 114, 116, 118, 121
    Handstand Rear Entry, 124
    Man on Top, 115–116, 133, 143
    Modified Missionary with Elevated Hips, 97
    orgasms and, 94, 95, 97, 114
    Peepshow, 122
    Pick-Me-Up, 127
    Pinwheel, 121
    postpartum sex, 40
    pregnancy and, 39–40
    Rear Entry, 97, 118, 129, 133, 144
    Reverse Cowgirl, 117, 133
    shower positions, 130
    Sitting, 121
    Spooning, 118, 143
    Standing Rear Entry, 118, 130
    Thigh Master, 124, 126
    view and, 114, 117, 122, 143
    Woman on Top, 97, 116–117, 130, 133, 144, 167
postpartum sex, 40–41, 43
preejaculatory fluid, 25, 103, 105, 106
pregnancy. See also birth control.
    abstinence and, 40
    anal play and, 39
    breasts and, 14
    communication and, 39
    endometrium and, 20
    forties and, 48
    genitals and, 38–39
    Kegel exercises and, 43
    normalization of, 11

oral sex and, 39
orgasms and, 43
physical changes and, 39, 43
Pinwheel position, 121
positions and, 39–40, 116, 118
postpartum birth control, 41
postpartum sex, 40–41, 43
preejaculatory fluid and, 103
Rear Entry position, 118
safety and, 39
semen and, 105
sex drive and, 38, 39, 44–45
Spooning position, 118
Thigh Master position, 124
uterus and, 20
Woman on Top position, 116
prepuce, 18
prolactin, 14
prostate stimulators, 169
P-spot, 103
puberty, 34–35
pubic mound. *See* mons.

Rabbit vibrator, 165
Rear Entry position, 97, 118, 129, 133, 144
Reverse Cowgirl position, 117, 133

Screaming O Vibrating Cock Ring, 169
Secretary, The (film), 183
serotonin, 74, 76
seventies, sex in, 52–53
sex-positive therapists, 10
sex toys
    anal play and, 139, 144, 165, 168
    BDSM, 182
    blindfolds, 182
    Bootie Silicone Anal Plug, 168
    Charm Silicone Dildo, 167
    clitoris and, 164, 165
    clothing, 183
    cock rings, 169
    communication and, 166
    condoms and, 139, 165, 169
    crops, 182
    dildos, 167, 168
    floggers, 182
    full-body restraints, 182
    G-spot and, 165, 167
    handcuffs, 182
    Hitachi Magic Wand, 165
    hygiene and, 165, 169
    lubrication and, 168
    male intimidation and, 166
    male sex toys, 165, 166, 169
    masturbation and, 65
    motivations for, 164–165
    orgasms and, 164
    porn and, 173
    prostate stimulators, 169
    Rabbit, 165
    safety, 169

Screaming O Vibrating Cock Ring, 169
    shopping for, 171
    suction-cup dildos, 167
    toxicity of, 169
    vibrators, 165, 168
    whips, 182
    wrist restraints, 182
"Sexual Behavior of the Human Male" (Alfred
    Kinsey), 175
sexual life spans
    twenties, 36, 38
    thirties, 43–45
    forties, 43–45, 48–49
    fifties, 49–50
    sixties, 51–52
    seventies, 52–53
sexually transmitted infections (STIs)
    blow jobs and, 105
    chlamydia, 28, 38, 105, 160
    communication and, 68
    condom misuse and, 27
    cunnilingus and, 160
    erectile disfunction and, 110
    fifties and, 49
    forties and, 48
    genital herpes, 29, 105, 160
    gonorrhea, 28, 38, 105, 160
    HIV/AIDS, 29, 105, 147
    hormonal birth control and, 25
    human papilloma virus (HPV), 29, 160
    preejaculatory fluid and, 105
    prevalence of, 35, 38, 49
    prevention of, 24, 38
    semen and, 105
    syphilis, 28, 160
    twenties and, 38
sexual orientation, 176
sexual self-esteem
    childhood and, 55–56
    communication and, 60, 68
    comparisons and, 59
    definition of, 56
    exercise and, 59
    masturbation, 61, 64–65
    plastic surgery and, 67
    practice and, 60
    questionnaire, 57
    regret and, 57
    role models, 59
    self-compliments and, 59
    sexual IQ and, 60
    "slut shaming," 59
    strengths and weaknesses, 59
shower sex, 130, 165, 167
Sinclair Institute website, 60
Sitting position, 121
sixties, sex in, 51–52
69 position, 160
Skene's glands, 94
sperm, 25, 27, 100, 103
Spooning position, 118, 143

Standing Rear Entry position, 118, 130
Sternberg, Robert, 77
Story of O, The (film), 183
Strano, Jackie, 144, 172
suction-cup dildos, 167
swinging, 178
syphilis, 28, 160

testosterone, 43, 45, 76
Thigh Master position, 124, 126
thirties, sex in, 43–45
threesomes, 177–178
toys. *See* sex toys.
Toys in Babeland website, 171
triangular theory of love, 77
trichinosis, 28
twenties, sex in, 36, 38

urethra
    female, 18, 19, 22, 28
    male, 100, 103, 106
urinary meatus, 18, 19
urinary tract infections (UTIs), 28, 48
uterus, 20, 39, 88

vagina
    anatomy texts and, 18
    depth of, 20, 103
    estrogen and, 76
    familiarization with, 11, 23
    location of, 20
    medical issues, 28–29
    orgasms and, 91
    vaginismus, 28, 97
    wall thickness, 45
vasopressin, 75, 76
Vaziri, Mo, 39, 44
Vex, Ulorin, 181
vibrators, 165, 168
virginity, loss of, 19, 35
vulva, 18–19

websites
    fatalemedia.com, 144
    Good Vibrations, 171
    Pleasure Chest, The, 171
    Sinclair Institute, 60
    swingers, 178
    Toys in Babeland, 171
Westheimer, Ruth, 43
Woman on Top position
    anal play and, 144
    car sex and, 133
    orgasms and, 97
    overview of, 116–117
    shower sex and, 130
    suction-cup dildos and, 167

yeast infections, 28, 48

About the Author

Amie Harwick is a marriage and family therapist in Los Angeles. Amie obtained her bachelor of arts in psychology from California Polytechnic University, Pomona, and her masters in clinical psychology from Pepperdine University. Her primary therapeutic focus is in areas surrounding sexuality with an emphasis on education to promote positive sexuality to reduce shame, and encouraging sexual self-awareness and personal growth. Amie writes for a variety of publications including *Playboy*, *Elite Daily*, and *Viva Glam Magazine*. Additionally, she has been showcased as an expert on current therapy issues with Fox News.

Acknowledgments

This book would have not been possible without the support and encouragement of those around me that have nurtured my quest for education, my desire to educate others, and my hope for social and cultural insight and awareness.

For their tolerance of late night calls and emails about proofreading, grammar, and insight, I want to thank my parents.

My gracious gratitude towards Moushumi Ghose for being an exceptional supervisor, mentor, and friend, and for helping me see possibilities and hope.

My sincere amazement and gratitude goes to everyone at Quiver Books for giving me the opportunity to write this book and for helping me to create a platform to continue to educate about sexuality. I want to specifically highlight the guidance and encouragement that Jill Alexander gave me throughout the process of the proposal, writing, and editing. My development editor, Megan Buckley, took the fear out of the editing process and made it a smooth and enlightening experience.

For introducing me to Quiver and shooting the beautiful images in the book, I want to express my appreciation to Holly Randall for her thoughtful connections and artistic talents.

For the comprehensive education, guidance from accomplished professors, and supporting me through my education and post-graduation career, I want to thank Pepperdine University.

I want to thank and acknowledge all of the people that gave me quotes for the book and opened up to me about their experiences, challenges, and desires.

Last, but not least, I want to thank my clients. They may not know that I have received and grown as much as them as they have from working with me.

Also Available

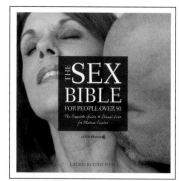

The Sex Bible For People Over 50
978-1-59233-500-8

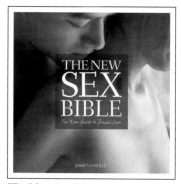

The New Sex Bible
978-1-59233-603-6

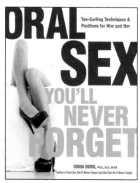

Oral Sex You'll Never Forget
978-1-59233-593-0

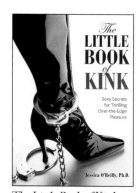

The Little Book of Kink
978-1-59233-574-9